Advance Praise for *Bad Boy*.

"The new edition of Donald Black's *Bad Boys, Bad Men* should be front and center on every thinking person's bookshelf. What makes antisocial personalities, psychopaths, and sociopaths tick? How did they get that way? Are they merely criminals who have no respect for the law, or do they have brain disorders that might benefit from treatment? I can think of no better source of expert and authoritative information to answer these questions than Black's new book. And there's a plus: Black is a good writer, and the book is filled with engrossing stories about real people with these conditions and what happened to them over time. A valuable book, and one that's hard to put down!"

—**John M. Oldham, MD,** *Senior Vice President and Chief of Staff, The Menninger Clinic; Professor and Executive Vice Chair, Menninger Department of Psychiatry and Behavioral Sciences, Baylor College of Medicine, Houston, TX*

"With this superb new volume, Donald Black has managed to produce an authoritative book on antisocial personality disorder and psychopathy that promises to be a valuable resource for partners and families of those touched by this disorder. In an accessible and jargon-free prose style that is a pleasure to read, the author describes the clinical picture, the causes, the outcomes, and potential treatments of antisocial individuals. He also educates the public on the so-called 'white collar sociopaths' who are hiding in plain sight. Mental health and medical professionals will gain as much from reading this outstanding contribution as the general public. I heartily recommend it."

—**Glen O. Gabbard, MD,** *Clinical Professor of Psychiatry, Baylor College of Medicine, Houston, TX*

BAD BOYS, BAD MEN

BAD BOYS, BAD MEN

Confronting
Antisocial Personality Disorder (*Sociopathy*)

Revised and Updated

Donald W. Black, MD

DEPARTMENT OF PSYCHIATRY
UNIVERSITY OF IOWA CARVER COLLEGE OF MEDICINE
IOWA CITY, IA

OXFORD
UNIVERSITY PRESS

OXFORD
UNIVERSITY PRESS

Oxford University Press is a department of the University of Oxford.
It furthers the University's objective of excellence in research, scholarship,
and education by publishing worldwide.

Oxford   New York

Auckland   Cape Town   Dar es Salaam   Hong Kong   Karachi
Kuala Lumpur   Madrid   Melbourne   Mexico City   Nairobi
New Delhi   Shanghai   Taipei   Toronto

With offices in

Argentina   Austria   Brazil   Chile   CzechRepublic   France   Greece
Guatemala   Hungary   Italy   Japan   Poland   Portugal   Singapore
South Korea   Switzerland   Thailand   Turkey   Ukraine   Vietnam

Oxford is a registered trade mark of Oxford University Press in the UK and certain other
countries.

Published in the United States of America by
Oxford University Press
198 Madison Avenue, New York, NY 10016

© Oxford University Press 2013

Library of Congress Cataloging-in-Publication Data
Black, Donald W., 1956–
Bad boys, bad men : confronting antisocial personality
disorder (sociopathy) / Donald W. Black.—2nd ed., rev. and updated. p. ; cm.
Includes bibliographical references and index.
ISBN 978-0-19-986203-0 (pbk)
I. Title.
[DNLM: 1. Antisocial Personality Disorder.   2. Men—psychology. WM 190.5.A2]
616.85'82—dc23 2012025162

The science of medicine is a rapidly changing field. As new research and clinical experience broaden our
knowledge, changes in treatment and drug therapy occur. The author and publisher of this work have
checked with sources believed to be reliable in their efforts to provide information that is accurate and
complete, and in accordance with the standards accepted at the time of publication. However, in light of
the possibility of human error or changes in the practice of medicine, neither the author, nor the publisher,
nor any other party who has been involved in the preparation or publication of this work warrants that the
information contained herein is in every respect accurate or complete. Readers are encouraged to confirm
the information contained herein with other reliable sources, and are strongly advised to check the product
information sheet provided by the pharmaceutical company for each drug they plan to administer.

1 3 5 7 9 8 6 4 2
Printed in the United States of America on acid-free paper

To the memory of the late George Winokur,
my friend and mentor

CONTENTS

PREFACE TO THE SECOND EDITION

Much has happened since this book was first published. The country has engaged in wars with Iraq and Afghanistan; Osama bin Laden was killed by Seal Team Six; the economy collapsed in 2008; and the Arab Spring brought unexpected surprises in the Middle East, not all of them good. And much has happened with antisocial personality disorder, or ASP, the acronym I use throughout this book. Data have accumulated regarding its prevalence and gender gap, possible causative factors (brain imaging and molecular genetics are hot topics these days), and new approaches to treatment. With all that has happened, I thought it was the right time to revise and update the book. Any reader who has written a book will understand my interest in writing a second edition. It presents an opportunity to make corrections, to edit or delete awkwardly written sentences (or paragraphs), and to include new material. It also gives the writer an opportunity to reflect on mountains of correspondence one has received.

In the past 13 years, as I'm sure is true for many authors, I have received a steady stream of letters and comments. People have purchased or borrowed the book for many reasons, and some are motivated to write (letters, emails) or phone to share their thoughts, insights, hopes, and dreams. Some just wanted to share sad stories from their true-life experience. And, yes, I have received my share of critical comments. I am grateful to all, including my critics, for taking the time to open their lives to me or, in the case of critical commentary, to force me to rethink what I had written and to address topics where, with reflection, I agree they may have a point. I also had my share of media interviews, some prompted by very real events, such as the shootings at Columbine High School in 1999. First, let me describe the positive feedback.

A few weeks after the book came out, I took a call from a physician in Des Moines. She was seeking my advice but, in truth, I believe she just wanted to talk. Her son had been difficult since age two and, now a man of 27, he continued to get into trouble with the law and was, at the time, sitting in the county jail awaiting trial. He had been in trouble all his life and as a teenager had ended up in juvenile detention. He had never been married, but had at least two children he was not supporting and a string of ex-girlfriends. Because of his temper and size, she was afraid of him. She had tried to do everything right, so she wondered how had she failed so miserably. I was at a loss for words.

Letters and emails began to arrive with similar themes, from wives, ex-wives, girlfriends, siblings, and so on. What was apparent was that most of my correspondence was from the women whose lives were ill-affected by someone who, to my ears, sounded anti-social. I then started to (and still do) receive letters from the men themselves, often prisoners. They shared their lives of woe and how they see themselves in my book. One of my research subjects, not portrayed in the book, called and asked to meet with me. I agreed to see him a few weeks later. He had brought a copy of my book, heavily marked up, and he wanted to share sections with me that were meaningful to him. He knew he had been "bad" but wanted to show me that he had improved and done his best to right the many wrongs committed earlier in life. In fact, he had worked as a chaplain for years at an Iowa prison. I believed him.

I also learned that, when writing a book, there are some people who will never be happy with either how the book is written or what is said. Some did not like my message and felt that ASP was a made-up condition. Others felt that I was sexist because I had not included women in my discussion or that I confused *psychopathy* with antisocial personality disorder. In response, I have enhanced the discussion of women antisocials and clarified the distinction between ASP and psychopathy. Some felt that my advice to antisocials themselves, in Chapter 10, was naïve. Yet I received positive feedback from family members and more than a few antisocial men themselves who agreed with my advice. Should I not encourage antisocials to make needed change?

I have aimed to make this book accessible to lay readers, yet scientifically responsible. Every major statement is backed up by scientific reports or opinions that can be found in the Notes section. For those seeking additional material, I have recommended a selection of books that I believe add, in a positive way, to furthering the discussion on ASP. The list is not comprehensive, and there are some books that probably should have been included but weren't. To those authors, I apologize in advance.

ACKNOWLEDGMENTS

The idea for this book came to me more than 20 years ago when I began my work with antisocial men. None of the books on antisocial personality disorder (ASP) was suitable for the general public except Hervey Cleckley's *The Mask of Sanity*, out of print since 1976. His book remains compelling reading, but much has happened since it was first published in 1941, including the seminal research that has defined ASP as we now know it.

In studying antisocial men, my research team and I collected an enormous amount of data. As the project came to a close, I wrote several manuscripts for medical journals. After submitting them for review, I was told by one respected but now deceased editor of a major journal that the papers contained too many "chatty" anecdotes and were not written in the "concise, bullet-like language" of scientific journals. I gave a spirited defense and replied that scientific journals are typically dull, as well as inaccessible to the lay person. I was unapologetic for writing interesting manuscripts. The response backfired, and perhaps I was overly defensive about my work. A kind man, he suggested I consider writing a book. The idea took form, and I later put into writing thoughts and ideas that had been on my mind for many years. With *Bad Boys, Bad Men,* my goal has been to educate lay readers and mental health professionals about a serious yet under-appreciated public health problem, and to help people with ASP and those whose lives have been negatively affected by them.

I am grateful to the many people who helped me write this book. The late George Winokur, former head of psychiatry at the University of Iowa, provided enormous guidance, from my initial conception of the book through the actual writing. I am indebted to my colleagues, the late Remi Cadoret, and Raymond Crowe, for their pioneering genetic research on ASP. My interactions with them over the years were of tremendous influence. My colleague Bruce Pfohl was a pioneer in the assessment of personality disorders. From him, I learned that these disorders were important and merited serious attention. (When I began my psychiatric training, these disorders were often trivialized or ignored altogether.) Nancy Andreasen, colleague and friend, taught me that there is no reason why science should be dry and unpalatable, as her books *The Broken Brain* and *Brave New Brain* amply demonstrate.

I am also thankful to the many friends and colleagues who read early drafts of the material. Their feedback was of enormous help. They include Peggy Baker, John Chadima, Ric Devor, Janelle Gabel, Chris Okiishi, Miriam Righter, Barb Rohland, Martha Shaw, Mary Webster, and Betty Winokur. Lin Larson, a talented writer and friend, helped organize and shape the manuscript. Liz Smothers, with her usual resourcefulness, deserves special thanks for assembling the photos and other illustrations.

Sue Ellen Bell and Cathy Butler (a pseudonym) merit special recognition. In their role as researchers, they were largely responsible for finding and interviewing the men profiled in this book. I am grateful to them for their ingenuity, persistence, and presence of mind. They were able to find people I thought untraceable, and they collected the many interesting nuggets that appear throughout the book.

ACKNOWLEDGMENTS

I am grateful to the men who opened up their lives to us and let us ask the most intimate of questions. Without their participation, the book could never have been written. I also wish to thank the countless patients I've worked with at the University of Iowa Hospitals and Clinics. They've taught me much of what I know about their disorders. They are the true teachers.

I am indebted to the staff at Oxford University Press, who have provided needed encouragement and technical support, in particular, editors Jeff House, who shared my vision for the book and helped give it form, and Craig Panner, who approached me about writing this update. We know a great deal more about ASP in 2012, and I felt it was time to revisit the disorder and take up where I had left off in 1999.

INTRODUCTION

It's normal to break the rules occasionally. Every day, many of us push the boundaries of what's permitted by social expectations and law. We engage in petty infractions likely to escape notice—taking long lunch breaks, inflating our accomplishments, driving too fast, or fibbing to family and friends. Some of us carry out larger, more dangerous schemes—cheating on spouses or partners, shoplifting, attempting to conceal a pattern of drug or alcohol abuse, and so on. Our offenses sometimes come back to haunt us and, through experience, most of us realize that the rules governing our daily lives have a purpose, even though we may never completely suppress the tendency to test their limits. Rules help maintain social order and protect each of us from harm. They help us live together as members of families and communities. Our entire lives are spent learning these rules and the benefits of conforming to them.

But some people never learn. From childhood on, they rebel against every type of regulation and expectation, seemingly oblivious to the value of living within society's boundaries. Despite all sanctions—parental punishment, ostracism, failure, or jail—they remain stuck in a rut of bad behavior, a rut they spend years digging without a second thought, and a rut that only gets deeper with time. Their resistance to authority and norms becomes the dominant force in their lives, often consigning them and their families to poverty, loneliness, addiction, and despair.

Many of us know someone who fits this description, at least to some degree. We may have relatives, friends, or neighbors who seem to be perpetually unemployed or in trouble with the law. Or we may know others whose words drip with dishonesty, hinting at a shady life behind a façade of respectability. Even those of us who don't know such people firsthand likely have encountered them in news reports of crime, poverty, and abuse. The chronic disregard for laws and social rules these people share is far more serious than the ordinary misdeeds most of us experience. Even those who commit isolated acts of serious misbehavior often realize their mistakes. Not so with those individuals whose lives run against the grain of society. At their mental and emotional core, many of these people don't seem to understand or care about the difference between good and bad, right and wrong.

Antisocial personality disorder, or ASP, is the term psychiatrists and other mental health professionals use to describe these people and their condition. Although many people know others who show signs of ASP, relatively few realize that a lifelong pattern of bad behavior is considered a mental disorder. In fact, psychiatry has wrestled with the problem of chronic antisocial behavior since the field began to take shape. This book describes much of what has been learned about ASP and traces the continuing search for answers. It also explores the possibility that ASP may be at the root of a substantial amount of the troubles that plague society, and that learning more about the disorder might help us fight crime, violence, and other social ills.

Perhaps the best, most concise definition of ASP comes from psychiatrists Donald Goodwin and Samuel Guze, in their book *Psychiatric Diagnosis*: "Sociopathy (sociopathic personality or antisocial personality) is a pattern of recurrent antisocial, delinquent, or criminal behavior that begins in early childhood or early adolescence and is manifested by disturbances in many areas of life: family relations, schooling, work, military service, and marriage."[1] The diagnosis of ASP relies on a mental health professional's ability to uncover this pattern and trace it through a patient's life. Isolated misdeeds or those confined to one area of life—work, for instance—are not by themselves evidence of ASP, although they may be the first clues to an underlying pattern of antisocial acts and attitudes.

Isolated misdeeds or misbehaviors are common and affect most of us at some point in our lives, but that does not indicate a diagnosis of ASP. Instead, the disorder is characterized by a *recurrent* and *serial* pattern of misbehavior that involves all significant facets of life and is marked by violation of social norms and regulations that occur over time, ranging from repeated lies and petty theft to violence—and even murder, in the most serious cases. The disorder's unpredictable range of expressions may sometimes lead to misdiagnosis because it is either explained away as a one-time occurrence, as the result of a chaotic upbringing, or as a predictable response to abuse. In truth, the diagnosis of ASP rests on the basis of the range and extent of antisocial acts over time, relying heavily on individual history.

It is important to note that in a psychiatric context, *antisocial* has nothing to do with a person's ability to socialize and is not used to describe those who are shy, inhibited, reclusive, or withdrawn. Rather, it implies a rebellion against society, a denial of the obligations that tie individuals to one another. People with ASP can be expertly social, adept at manipulating others when it serves their purposes, but their relationships often tend to be superficial, short-lived, and bereft of trust. I use the word *antisocial* (or *antisocials*) when referring to people with the disorder, but the older term *sociopath* is probably used even more often in the lay media and may be more familiar to readers. *Psychopath* is an even more chilling word, but, as I discuss in Chapter 3, the term has a particular meaning that does not fully overlap with ASP.

An especially troubling aspect of ASP is that many, perhaps the majority, of antisocials seem to lack a conscience, feeling little or no empathy for the people whose lives they touch.[2] This emotional aloofness is what potentially makes the antisocial so dangerous. For those lacking a conscience, anything goes, including the most vicious crimes—crimes that may be repeated again and again, with no concern for their victims. It is as if a vital part of the antisocial's character—his moral compass—is somehow absent or underdeveloped. This essential part of our humanity makes us adhere to social rules and obligations. Freed from the constraint of conscience, some antisocials effortlessly resist all regulation, unable to see beyond their own self-interest or to adopt standards of right versus wrong. In her book *The Stranger Beside Me*, Ann Rule writes that serial killer Ted Bundy went through life without a conscience, which she describes as the "factor that separates us from animals. It allows us to love, to feel another's pain, and to grow. Whatever the drawbacks are to being blessed with a conscience, the rewards are essential to living in a world with other human beings. [The] psychopath might as well be a visitor from another planet, struggling to mimic the feelings of those he encounters."[3] By way of analogy, consider the color-blind man unable to distinguish red from green: He knows the colors exist, but cannot distinguish them. Here, too, like Bundy, the person lacking a conscience may understand the concept and understand he is different from others, but he is unable to internalize those feelings we call remorse.

This book's title, as well as my repeated use of the masculine when talking about antisocials, reflects the fact that, for practical purposes, ASP is a disorder of men. It is up to eight times more common in men than women. (The precise ratio of men to women is unknown, but the figure tends to vary from study to study.) In addition, my own research study, described in Chapter 1 and which forms the basis of the book, focused entirely on men for the simple reason that we had trouble finding antisocial women who fit the criteria. Clearly, women *do* develop the disorder, but their symptoms may be less outwardly directed and tend not to feature the alarming spasms of crime or violence so characteristic of male antisocials. The modern definition of ASP is another factor that may be involved, because it reflects behavior patterns more frequently observed among men. For that reason, related symptoms exhibited by women are commonly regarded as signs of different psychiatric disorders, for example *borderline personality disorder* which, as I will show, is fundamentally different from ASP. That said, as an equal opportunity disorder, the woman antisocial, like the man, is troublesome to her family and community, and some are fully capable of showing a disturbing degree of violence. I will take up the antisocial woman and describe what sets her apart from men later in the book.

The ignorance that surrounds ASP reflects its complexity. Antisocial personality disorder and other personality disorders confound the common understanding of mental illness because they generally do not spawn psychosis, blur one's perception of reality, induce paralyzing emotional states, or constitute legal insanity. They are sometimes described as character disorders, for they denote deep flaws in one's perception of self and of one's place in the world. Psychiatrists and psychologists have observed, defined, and attempted to treat *personality disorders* for many years, but some might still argue that they are not legitimate psychiatric conditions or are, at the very least, less legitimate disorders than, say, schizophrenia or bipolar disorder. In the case of ASP, critics have warned that the "medicalization" of antisocial behavior risks excusing immorality by labeling it a disease. They argue that bad behavior stems from poor judgment, moral apathy, or social and spiritual deficits beyond the scope of medicine.

These complaints misunderstand ASP and disregard growing evidence that many aspects of personality and behavior can be traced to the workings of brain and body. An ASP diagnosis is not a license for patients to behave as they like, but instead is a lens through which to view their misbehavior, which is unusual by any standard. We notice antisocials because they stand apart from the norm. The evolution of ASP as a psychiatric diagnosis has been in part an effort to understand why antisocials turn out the way they do, why they cause so many serious problems that cannot be ignored. Although ASP holds many mysteries, strong evidence links it to heredity, brain injury, body chemistry, and other medical factors. But the inquiry into ASP raises difficult questions: Where does the self come from? Are our individual personalities products of our genes? Can we undo the work of genetic or environmental forces that shape who we are? Although these existential questions are beyond the scope of this book, I do hope to offer a background that will help readers reach their own conclusions.

Chapter 1 briefly recounts my early experience with ASP and describes its occurrence throughout society, even when it goes unrecognized. Chapter 2 traces the history of efforts to understand ASP and the development of modern diagnostic criteria for the disorder. Chapter 3 outlines its symptoms, including the link between childhood and adult misbehavior that renders ASP a lifelong problem, and the special features that mark the antisocial woman. The process of diagnosis is explained in Chapter 4, followed by a discussion of ASP's course and outcome in Chapter 5. Chapter 6 probes suspected causes of the disorder, which seem to stem from a complex interplay of genetics and environment. In Chapter 7, I discuss current treatment recommendations for ASP and the other disorders that frequently accompany it. Chapter 8 looks at antisocials who manage to make their way in society, often by suspicious means. Chapter 9 focuses on serial killer and study subject John Wayne Gacy, exploring what can happen when ASP reaches its worst potential. Chapter 10 provides advice to antisocials and families coping with the disorder.

We can all benefit from understanding ASP and its effects on individuals and families, learning to see it when it appears in our culture and our daily lives. I've written this book to explain ASP in language that a general audience can understand, and I have tried to show how this complex disorder appears before us almost every day. Although I suspect few antisocials will read the book or recognize themselves in its pages, I hope some may find it helpful in gaining a better understanding of their condition. For family members, friends, and relatives of antisocials, this book has been written as a resource that explains the disorder and aims to help them deal with its consequences. People in the helping professions—physicians, nurses, social workers, mental health providers, lawyers—who work with antisocials daily have a pressing need for more information about the disorder, and victims of crime and abuse may find here a better understanding of those who have hurt them.

Nearly everyone has a friend, colleague, relative, or acquaintance whose life is touched by ASP. The disorder is so common that *not* to know an antisocial is itself remarkable. The closer one is to the disorder, the more one knows about its destructive potential, but even those who do not experience it firsthand pay for ASP in one way or another—whether in dollars or in fear. Research into ASP is an unfinished project that receives little popular or financial support, but it remains a necessary step toward achieving understanding. Perhaps when we unlock the secrets of ASP, we will discover the roots of many problems that continue to bedevil society.

Readers should know that not all the examples of bad behavior appearing in this book involve people with ASP. Because ASP is characterized by a pattern of socially irresponsible, exploitive, and guiltless behavior, the diagnosis is generally viewed as pejorative and potentially stigmatizing. It ought never to be used lightly or in a way that trivializes its importance. Although all cases from my own work have been carefully diagnosed based on extensive files and interviews, other persons described in this book, both famous and infamous, have not been diagnosed as antisocial. Their stories are used to illustrate aspects of antisocial behavior. A person should not be assumed to have ASP simply because he or she is mentioned in this book.

BAD BOYS, BAD MEN

Chapter 1

A Lurking Threat

Antisocial Personality Disorder and Society

THE PROBLEM EMERGES

At first, she tried to look beyond his bad habits—the nights he spent out drinking while she lay awake at home, the snarling insults that punctuated arguments, the tendency to throw things or punch walls. Tom's life had been tough, she reminded herself, and he was just out of prison after serving a sentence for armed robbery, a sentence cut short by good behavior. In time, he would get a job, simmer down, and settle into the life she imagined for them. She focused on his better side—his charm and promises, good looks, and other traits she thought she remembered from the first weeks of their relationship. But things gradually grew worse, and eventually no fond memories could counter the reality of the moment. One evening, she made dinner, set the table with her grandmother's dishes, and asked him to please stay home. He brushed aside her request, but she persisted. Finally, he upended the table in a fit of rage, littering the floor with pot roast, mashed potatoes, and fragments of china. Terrified, Tom's girlfriend managed to stand her ground, issuing a tearful ultimatum: Get help or lose her.

Tom's temper was explosive and unpredictable, unusual in its intensity and hair-trigger nature. I know because I was the psychiatry resident assigned to care for him when he came to the hospital at his girlfriend's insistence. During my months of training on the ward, I had worked with all types of patients and thought I had seen just about everything: catatonics who neither spoke nor moved; schizophrenics who heard secret voices or shared whispers with the Devil; men and women mired in depression, longing for death; anorexic girls slowly starving themselves. But Tom was different.

He was pleasant enough during our first meeting, cooperating as I performed the mental status examination, a routine then new to me. After correctly identifying the date, his location, and the reason for his hospitalization, Tom moved effortlessly through the series of questions designed to assess memory and mental functions. He denied being depressed or anxious, or using drugs, and smirked when I asked about voices, hallucinations, and paranoia. As my questions persisted ("Do you ever get special messages over the TV?") he began to lose his patience, and I could hear the first rumblings of anger behind his answers. The test revealed no apparent signs of a major psychiatric illness.

A physical examination told me even less. Tom was tall and sinewy, his body strengthened by hours in the prison recreation room. An elaborate skull and crossbones tattoo decorated his muscular shoulder, in contrast to the crude heart and initials tattooed into his left hand with India ink and a needle—his own work, he noted. I ordered the standard blood and urine tests, as well as an electroencephalographic tracing of his brain waves after he told me about a childhood head injury. The normal results excluded a range of medical causes for his violent temper. Further psychological tests confirmed my opinion that there was no evidence of depression, anxiety, or psychosis.

But Tom clearly was not normal. My interviews with him revealed a life of early abuse, violence, and crime. One of five children born to a depressed mother and an alcoholic father, Tom weathered years of beatings and neglect. He learned to steal while young, snatching money from his mother's purse before moving on to neighbors' homes and nearby businesses. Adolescence brought experiments with drugs and sex, regular drinks with older boys, and an unplanned pregnancy aborted by his teenage girlfriend. His dismal performance at school ended when he was expelled for setting fire to a restroom.

As Tom grew up, his exploits became more daring, violent, and difficult to ignore. Arrested frequently for breaking and entering, robbery, and fighting, Tom rambled through his teen years without any sense of direction. Girlfriends came and went, at first drawn to his sly good looks and tough physique, then driven away by his unpredictable rage and jealousy, which sometimes erupted in sexual violence. Eventually, his record caught up with him, and he was sent to prison on the armed robbery charge that preceded his hospitalization.

Four days after he entered the hospital, I was ready to let him go. The early charm he had shown dissolved into bickering, threats, and absurd demands. He argued constantly, cajoled a night aide into loaning him cigarette money, hosted a parade of unkempt visitors, and demanded special passes to see his girlfriend. After I refused to prescribe tranquilizers for his newly self-diagnosed anxiety, he made ambiguous threats of a malpractice suit. In fact, Tom snubbed every effort to treat him, showing no interest in the source of his anger or any means to control it. He greeted my every word with the same bored stare and dominated group therapy with rants about how others—his girlfriend, parents, neighbors, doctors, and just about everyone else—were responsible for all his problems. He argued that the hospital would do him no good, and after a while, I found myself agreeing with him.

Frustrated by Tom's behavior and my inability to reach him, I consulted with my supervisor, a seasoned clinician, who patiently listened to my concerns and then suggested a discharge. Tom was a sociopath, he said, and there was no treatment for his condition. He would resist all my efforts and seek to exploit those around him. There was nothing I could do. The discussion did little to relieve my frustration, and I felt no satisfaction when Tom was finally discharged after repeatedly refusing counseling.

Over the course of my residency, I met other men like Tom. All shared the history of erratic, irresponsible, and often violent behavior that characterizes antisocial personality disorder (ASP). Although I came to understand the diagnosis through my experiences with these men, ASP remained for me a source of fascination and perplexity. I could not understand the total self-absorption these men exhibited, their failure to accept responsibility for their actions, their facile explanations that defied credulity, and their almost total disregard for others. I couldn't help wondering why we tried to treat them. Most led miserable lives but continually failed to see how their actions contributed to their troubles, and every attempt at counseling ran up against their sheer inability to look inward. I was overwhelmed by their problems—depression, alcoholism, domestic violence, and a host of other ills—and felt inadequate in the face of their pathological defiance. What made it so difficult for them to live by any rule? What was I to do with these men?

After years of studying ASP and working with those affected by it, I still have many of these same questions. Antisocial personality disorder remains misunderstood, both within psychiatry and by society at large, its causes almost as elusive as its treatments. Yet it appears to be at least as common as other conditions that capture public attention, such as panic disorder, obsessive-compulsive disorder (OCD), and attention-deficit/hyperactivity disorder (ADHD). Among the major psychiatric illnesses, only depression occurs more frequently. In the recent National Epidemiologic Survey on Alcohol and Related Conditions (NESARC) study, a large-scale survey of psychiatric disorders among 43,000 Americans, about 3.6% of people interviewed—5.5% of men and 1.9% of women—were diagnosed antisocial.[1] By comparison, the figures were 13.2% for major depression, 5.1% for panic disorder, and 4.4% for ADHD. Other studies have shown that OCD has a prevalence of 1.6%, whereas schizophrenia occurs in about 1.5% of the population.

These ASP prevalence rates may sound remarkably high to those unfamiliar with the disorder. In fact, they may not be high enough, because many antisocials deny, forget, or frankly lie when questioned about their symptoms. I discovered this firsthand when I interviewed men whose antisocial history was fully documented and found that a quarter of them refused to admit past misbehavior.[2] Further, NESARC data do not include those in prisons or other institutions—nearly 2.3 million people in the United States—of whom many are antisocial.[3] Omitting these individuals from the prevalence estimates makes the disorder appear less common than it actually is.

That said, if the 3.6% figure cited in the NESARC is applied to the general population of the United States over age 18 years, a staggering 8.5 million Americans may be antisocial.[4] Whatever its actual prevalence, the nature of ASP implies that it wreaks more havoc on society than most other mental illnesses do, because the disorder primarily involves reactions against the social environment that drag other people into its destructive web. Many mental disorders have serious implications beyond patients and their families, such as lost productivity and treatment costs. But the social impact of ASP seems more immediate. Antisocial criminals are responsible for untold losses and require billions of dollars to police and punish them. The despair and anxiety wrought by antisocials tragically affect families and communities, leaving deep physical and emotional scars—especially on their children, who often grow up to follow their parents' difficult paths through life. Many antisocials live in poverty or draw on the social welfare system, hampered by poor school and work performance and an inability to establish a life plan. The costs—economic, social, and emotional—of ASP defy calculation, in part because the disorder's prevalence and impact remain uncertain.

But the true price of ASP is expressed in more subtle ways as well, including a diffuse sense of mistrust about the intentions of others. Crime and other social problems stem from a variety of causes in addition to ASP, but antisocials and their actions contribute to our collective fears and preoccupations. These fears drive us to quicken our steps on a dark street, to lock our cars and houses, to suspect others' promises. Although these instincts guard us from danger, they can become harmful if they convince us that nothing is safe, that society's rules no longer afford any protection or assurance of order. Today's concerns about crime, corruption, and social cohesion make this a good time to explore ASP and its role in the social problems we witness. Our interest in the roots of bad behavior should prompt us to take a closer look at this psychiatric disorder and its destructive manifestations.

A SECRET ALL AROUND US

There is a widespread sentiment that public life and moral standards in the United States are on the decline. Many Americans voice concern that the rules no longer seem to work, that society has lost its moral center, and that our culture needs to reclaim fundamental values (which vary, of course, depending on who is asked). Former Secretary of Education William Bennett's collection *The Book of Virtues* and its assorted offshoots and imitators have become national best-sellers.[5] Political rhetoric is peppered with calls for a return to "traditional values" and "personal responsibility"—qualities that some argue have been lost to a culture of permissiveness. Dubious rationales for bad behavior are condemned in books like Alan Dershowitz's *The Abuse Excuse and Other Cop-Outs, Sob Stories, and Evasions of Responsibility*, which documents efforts to blame misdeeds on everything from spousal battery to religious sentiments to premenstrual syndrome.[6]

It's hard to say whether this sense of decline is a response to true change or a media-induced notion that comes to life daily in our homes and work places. After all, we have learned over and over again "if it bleeds, it leads." Stories of teenagers abandoning babies in restrooms, students murdering their teachers, and habitual sex offenders raping children might once have been fodder for local newspapers. Today, they're beamed cross country on the evening news and are on the Internet 24/7. Few things raise a tremor in public consciousness like crime and violence, the most bizarre and brutal offenses drawing frenzied calls for action, however rare and unpredictable they may be. Elected representatives have responded to current concerns with escalating rhetoric about curbing violence through "get-tough" measures calculated more for their political expediency than for their potential to solve problems.[7] Candidates for office vow to build more prisons, lock up more criminals, stiffen penalties, stage more executions, and promote morality. Those who appear "soft" on crime, or to coddle criminals, or even to question the revolving door of our correctional system, are unlikely to be elected.

As a psychiatrist, trained to observe and interpret human behavior, I often see evidence of ASP where others see signs of amorphous social decay. The metaphorical lack of a moral center becomes literal in the blatant disregard for social regulation at the core of ASP. Knowledge of this condition may help explain acts that seem to defy interpretation and may also persuade us that some of the violence we see on the news and in the streets is endemic not to our culture, but rather to a group of individuals who share a serious disorder that receives scant attention.

Reports of high-profile violent crimes provide glimpses of people whose lives show some of the patterns associated with ASP. Although I don't profess to diagnose these individuals with ASP or any other disorder, I recognize in their histories many of my patients' characteristics. A closer look at some recent events illustrates what I mean by recurring patterns of antisocial behavior and attitudes traced through individual histories.

During the 1990s, the incessant media spectacle that surrounded O. J. Simpson's criminal and civil trials on the charge that he murdered his ex-wife, Nicole Brown Simpson, and her friend Ronald Goldman, made it one of the 20th century's best-known criminal cases. Simpson was found not guilty of the criminal murder charge but was later found liable for the deaths in civil court. His very public trials involved evidence of domestic abuse, rage, and pathological jealousy of an intensity rare even among antisocials. Simpson's life reveals a history of misbehavior that began during his early years in San

Francisco's tough Potrero Hill neighborhood.[8] Described as "rowdy" and a "half-bully who engaged in petty thievery and extortion," he had joined a gang by age 14. His teen years also included an arrest for stealing from a liquor store. After becoming a football and media superstar, Simpson was known for his sexual exploits, developed a drug problem, and narrowly escaped two separate drug busts. His first marriage was turbulent, and his second—to Nicole—brought a 1989 arrest for domestic battery, to which Simpson pleaded guilty and paid a $200 fine. A 1993 recording of a 911 call revealed after the murders demonstrates his capacity for rage, and photographs submitted as evidence showed a battered and bruised Nicole, allegedly beaten by Simpson. After their divorce, he reportedly stalked her, possessed by jealousy.

And the Simpson story is not over. Although shunned by all except his most rabid fans, he eventually moved to Florida (where a person's residence cannot be sold to collect a debt) and wrote what he described as a fictional account of the murders, called *If I Did It*. The book was later withdrawn by the publisher but, in an odd turn of fate, publication rights were acquired by the Goldman family from a Florida bankruptcy court, and it was published with a new subtitle: *Confessions of a Killer*. Following a series of minor legal skirmishes in Florida, Simpson was arrested and convicted of numerous felonies, including armed robbery and kidnapping stemming from a bizarre attempt to retrieve sports memorabilia at a Las Vegas hotel. Sentenced to 33 years in prison, he could be paroled as early as 2017. Despite the years of violence, and the pain of ostracism and financial ruin, O. J. seemed never to learn to conform to society's rules.

A more recent case that became a national obsession, and one that weaves together ASP and senseless violence, is that of Joran van der Sloot. The youthful and roguishly handsome van der Sloot became a suspect in the May 2005 disappearance of 18-year-old Natalee Holloway, a college student vacationing on the island of Aruba.[9]

Originally from Holland, he was considered a star athlete, but was dogged with rumors of lying and gambling. In a story with many twists and turns, van der Sloot was arrested as a suspect soon after Holloway's disappearance, but was released due to lack of evidence. He gave a series of contradictory media interviews, and even wrote a book to tell his side of the story. He lost all credibility when a Dutch journalist made an undercover video that showed van der Sloot smoking pot and admitting he was present at Holloway's death, although the courts deemed the evidence insufficient. In the meantime, he moved to Bangkok, where he bought a restaurant and was about to become involved in sex trafficking, using an alias to avoid the authorities. By then, he called himself a professional poker player. He returned to Aruba following his father's death in 2010 and was the subject of a sting operation after he offered to reveal the location of Natalee's body to a representative of the Holloway family for $250,000. He received an initial payment of $10,000 and promptly fled to Lima, Peru. In 2010, he pleaded guilty to the robbery and murder of a young woman who was savagely beaten to death exactly 5 years after the disappearance of Holloway. He was sentenced to 28 years in prison.

I offer these examples to show what many of us, even those who have never heard of ASP, already realize: People charged with brutal crimes often have a history of trouble, be it tied to family, other relationships, work, school, or the law. Although such histories cannot always be ascribed to ASP, they epitomize the lives lived by antisocials—lives that sometimes culminate in shocking acts of violence. To be fair, most of the acts committed by antisocials are less dramatic, involving deception, exploitation, and ruses ranging from comic to cruel. Most antisocials live quiet lives next door, down the block, or sometimes under the same roof, and their exploits are fodder for neither the local news outlet nor the tabloid culture.

Not all media portrayals of antisocial behavior are sensationalized accounts of violence. A *Des Moines Register* profile of one Paul

Mendez claimed to offer a "Portrait of a Real Hobo—Footloose, Fighting, Sometimes Bitter."[10] The story followed Mendez through a typical day of drinking and panhandling and, although it presented him as a contrast to the image of the carefree, happy-go-lucky hobo, the narrative retained a veiled respect for his rejection of authority and social convention: "Most of the time he's calm and smiling. He's mellowed with age.... He says that he used to steal, but doesn't now. He says he hasn't been in prison since 1978.... He stays at missions when he needs a shower, but he doesn't like to follow their rules." Mendez's history of criminality, drug abuse, and rootlessness; his dislike for regulation; and his somewhat unpredictable moods would support a diagnosis of ASP. Yet he is regarded by the reporter as harmless, having settled into the lifestyle that suits him, perhaps to be envied for his freedom from the responsibilities that many of us face.

The antisocial personality often has been embraced by popular culture as both a source of fear and an object of envy. Sometimes, we are fascinated by the deviousness, crudity, or cruelty of his crimes and misdeeds, perhaps drawn by a voyeuristic blend of curiosity and repulsion. At other times, we may be motivated by envy of his perceived freedom or defiant rejection of rules. Occasionally, we are entertained by his bizarre behavior—so long as it is harmless or distant enough. Interest in the antisocial may be especially strong in a culture that holds individual liberty in the highest esteem. The antisocial is the ultimate individualist, shirking responsibilities that many of us would never—and could never—consider abandoning. The myths obscure the fact that ASP is a pathological disorder that touches millions of lives in ways we seldom understand.

Although supermarket tabloids and lowbrow talk shows exploit antisocial traits for cheap entertainment, they have long been a staple of Hollywood. Many popular films and books celebrate the antisocial as attractive protagonists or compelling villains. Cary Grant plays a smooth con artist in Hitchcock's *Suspicion*, above all manner of social regulation. In *Rebel Without a Cause*, a title that connotes a romantic view of the antisocial, James Dean is the delinquent antihero, stifled by convention and rules. Even films that portray the antisocial personality as a menace, such as *Cape Fear*, *Silence of the Lambs*, or *The Talented Mr. Ripley*, often make him more central and captivating than other characters. Perhaps today's most visible antisocial is the eponymous *Dexter*. A brooding blood-spatter expert, *Dexter* hunts down and kills serial killers in his spare time. Instilled by his adoptive father, Dexter's "code" requires that he only use his dark force (that is, murderous urges) to do good.

The antisocial has a long history in literature, from Shakespeare's plays, to Dickens's novels of Victorian England, to Sinclair Lewis's indictments of 20th-century America. Across literary genres, antisocial characters appear again and again, here the subject of a true crime book, there profiled in a biography or psychological study.[11] Even commercial self-help books regularly deal with antisocial behavior. *Bad Boys: Why We Love Them, How to Live with Them, and When to Leave Them*, for example, offers advice to women who fall into relationships with men who arguably sound antisocial.[12]

The best depictions of antisocial personalities, real or imagined, strip away the veneer of romance to depict the conflict and destructive potential of their characters. One classic account, Truman Capote's *In Cold Blood*, explores the widely reported murder of a Kansas farm family in order to uncover the minds and motivations of the killers.[13] Mikal Gilmore's *Shot in the Heart* provides a moving insight into the family dynamics of ASP. The book traces antisocial behavior and its repercussions through two generations, from a sadistic, alcoholic father who beats his wife and children, cheats innocents out of their savings, and takes his family on the lam, to Gilmore's infamous brother Gary, executed for double murder in 1977.[14] The book's title refers to Gilmore's execution by a firing squad, a choice available then in Utah, influenced by the Mormon doctrine of blood atonement.

But antisocials are not just characters in our fictional or true-life entertainments. They are family members, friends, co-workers, neighbors, or strangers we may encounter every day. Their disorder is often difficult to hide, and some antisocials manage to keep it under wraps through elaborate cons, colorful lies, and brash attempts at charm. Sometimes, though, friends and family members become accomplices in antisocials' efforts to hide their nature. They pretend nothing is wrong while ignoring even the most outrageous behaviors, or they hold out hope that the problem will pass. Unfortunately, it seldom does. We have an astonishing capacity to overlook or forgive the faults of those close to us, from the friend who ran out on his wife and refuses to support his children, to the cousin jailed for forging checks, to the brother who deals drugs on the sly. That these people may be antisocial seldom enters the mind, even when their misdeeds assume obvious patterns and turn ever more destructive.

BEHAVIOR AND CONTEXT

Not all antisocial behavior points to ASP. Rather, a complex blend of actions and attitudes characterizes the disorder, and antisocial behavior must be judged in context when looking for clues to ASP. Familiar standards of right and wrong may fail under extreme circumstances that revise the rules of behavior. Different societies operate under different rules that make what's right in one cultural context wrong in another. Finally, isolated antisocial acts are common even among people who don't have ASP. Recognizing true cases of ASP requires an awareness of its context and an ability to discern far-ranging patterns of bad behavior.

Antisocial behavior becomes the norm in situations in which there are no more rules to be broken and what was once unthinkable becomes commonplace. War provides a dramatic example. In places like Iraq or Afghanistan, citizens have engaged in atrocities that would otherwise constitute grave violations of social norms or laws—destroying property, killing, raping. But in the context of war, these activities are sanctioned, however loosely, and probably cannot be seen as true manifestations of ASP, although they may be equally inexplicable.

Definitions of right and wrong also vary from culture to culture, and the specific behaviors that represent ASP vary as well. Some argue that because society sets the standard for behavior, authoritarian cultures with severe penalties for misdeeds are the most successful at controlling the antisocial impulse. Societies with little tolerance for violating social norms indeed may have low crime rates—like those of Saudi Arabia, where strict punishments are swiftly meted out, or Singapore, where chewing gum may be considered an antisocial act. These societies deal harshly with antisocial behavior when it reaches a certain threshold, but that doesn't mean they can control or eradicate ASP. The disorder appears to be universal. Cross-cultural studies that apply American criteria for ASP to places like Hong Kong, Korea, and New Zealand show ASP prevalence rates similar to those in the United States.[15]

Regardless of the historical or cultural context, isolated misbehaviors that defy social regulation are very common. In the Epidemiologic Catchment Area (ECA) study, a large survey of 15,000 Americans conducted in the early 1980s at five different sites, 30% of men surveyed in St. Louis reported four or more moving-traffic arrests, 18% admitted being unfaithful to their wives in three or more affairs, and 8% claimed to have held an illegal occupation, like drug dealing, at some point in their lives. Thirty-four percent of those surveyed in Baltimore had a history of isolated antisocial symptoms.[16] Based on these findings, at least one-quarter to one-third of the population has some history of antisocial behavior, although far fewer exhibit the severe and varied symptoms that justify a diagnosis of ASP. Knowing that so many of us flout the rules at some point in our lives may prevent us from recognizing those who live in constant defiance of norms and expectations and thus may contribute to the widespread misunderstanding of ASP. Too often, perhaps, we see the individual's antisocial acts as simple faults that many people share, not noticing patterns that set him apart from the healthy but imperfect norm.

Mental illness is frequently invoked as a rationale for crime, and attributing bad behavior to ASP may rouse debate in a time when excuses seem to proliferate faster than they can be debunked. Antisocial personality disorder, however, is no excuse and, in the United States, has only rarely been used as a legal defense.[17] Unlike some other psychiatric conditions—schizophrenia, for instance—it does not rob those who have it of the ability to distinguish right from wrong. Antisocials realize what their options are and can choose not to break the rules, commit crimes, or walk out on their responsibilities, but the problem is their constant failure to do so. Like most psychiatrists, I believe antisocials should be held fully responsible for their actions, and, over the years, I have informed many such individuals under my care of that as well. But it is not enough to say that people with ASP are simply "bad" or "immoral." Their unusual histories of misbehavior set them apart from others who engage in isolated or occasional antisocial acts, and the search for what makes them different may eventually shed light on mechanisms that govern much of human behavior.

THE NEED FOR KNOWLEDGE AND THE IOWA STUDY

Why is ASP, a common and costly psychiatric disorder and a major public health concern, largely ignored? In some cases, the diverse problems faced by antisocials—crime, spousal abuse, poor job performance, and the like—are never linked and traced to a common root because the pattern of misbehavior occurring over time is either ignored or has escaped attention. Antisocial personality disorder is often misdiagnosed because its true scope goes unrecognized, but other factors contribute to its low profile. Antisocials themselves can be uncooperative or even unpleasant to the doctors or therapists charged with their care, thus complicating efforts to study and treat them. Funding agencies that support psychiatric research channel little money to ASP studies, and this includes the National Institutes of Health.[18] Projects on the genetics of violence and other behavior problems related to ASP are politically sensitive, with some critics arguing that racial bias inevitably taints such work. Perhaps most important, there have been no breakthroughs in the treatment of ASP, and many mental health professionals consider it hopeless.

Early in my career, as a young psychiatric researcher, my initial decision to study ASP was partly a pragmatic effort to fill a gap in the literature. There were few outcome data on antisocials, making it a fertile area for me as I took up an academic career. I was also driven by personal interest. My experiences with men like Tom had raised important questions about the nature of the disorder and the challenge of treating it, questions that motivated me to investigate what happened to these men as they grew older—how they changed, and, if they had improved, what might have been responsible, and whether they improved at all. Following the model of a mentor, Dr. George Winokur, who had studied the course and outcome of bipolar (manic-depressive) disorder and schizophrenia, I decided to seek out men who had once been diagnosed antisocial, to discover what had become of them.[19] It was the beginning of a major project that required nearly as much detective work as science, and one that led to a lifelong interest in ASP.

To help with this journey, I relied on the efforts of two research assistants, Cathy Butler and Sue Ellen Bell. I began by examining the hospital records of antisocial men treated at the University of

Iowa Psychopathic Hospital (later changed to Psychiatric Hospital) between 1945 and 1970, many there because of a court order or urged by desperate family members to undergo psychiatric evaluation. My goal was to find the men, interview them, and compare their present situations to their past experiences and diagnoses.[20]

In the pre-Internet era, finding the men took enormous ingenuity and resolve. Today, one need only to enter a name for a Google search and the person's current location is often only a click away—to the surprise and dismay of many. Not so in the 1980s, when finding someone was a major challenge. Complicating our task was the fact that many antisocials assume new names and move frequently to escape their troubles. We tried using past addresses and phone numbers, called friends and family members who were listed in the charts, contacted government agencies, and used whatever other options seemed to produce clues. In one case, Cathy had almost given up on finding a subject until she noticed an entry in his chart that we had previously overlooked. It noted that the subject's father was dead, prompting Cathy to obtain a copy of his death certificate and contact the funeral director listed. The man remembered that our subject's sister had paid for the funeral, and he gave Cathy her phone number. With the sister's help, Cathy managed to reach the subject, only to have him refuse to take part!

To coax otherwise recalcitrant men to participate, we offered a modest $25. One subject was contacted in California, where he claimed to be mining for gold on the Trinity River. He later returned to Iowa and agreed to an interview at the Des Moines YMCA but was upset when told that he wouldn't be paid for two weeks. He needed the money, he said, for the start-up fee necessary to become a cab driver. Without it, he was flat broke, having carelessly spent a sizable inheritance during his 8 years on the West Coast. The compensation failed to sway others, however, including one who told Cathy to put her money "where the sun don't shine." He had been in jail for 9 years (a "bum rap," he said); he snorted that he could take care of himself, then slammed the phone down.

Family members of several men became valuable informants. One man's wife told us he was "very complicated," meaning he was a compulsive liar, con artist, and abusive spouse. He was trying to draw Social Security benefits under three different names, the latest in a lifelong series of scams that included lying his way into marriage. His wife had thought herself his first spouse but later learned he had been married twice before. Although he agreed to talk with us, he denied nearly everything she had reported—as well as most of the information on his official record. He had married just once, by his own account, had committed only one unidentified felony, and claimed to be a highly regarded engineer for a major car manufacturer.

Many of the men we talked to had no qualms about admitting their past and present misdeeds, even inflating them for our benefit. We knew that much of what we heard departed from the truth, but we simply considered a subject's lies further evidence that he had not improved. Our subjects were overwhelmingly white, blue collar, lower middle class, and married, and most had not graduated from high school. They had typically been in their 20s when hospitalized and were in their 50s when contacted for our study. (Our oldest subject was 79.) Most had long histories of bad behavior that had sometimes waned, and other times continued unabated. Few expressed shame or remorse for the trouble they had caused, nor did any seem especially embarrassed when relating their lies, cons, and wild schemes to us. Their stories make up much of this book and offer glimpses into the lives of men with ASP. Details are taken from case records and interview notes—true accounts presented without embellishment, although, in all but one case, names and other details have been changed to preserve confidentiality. They reveal the impact of this disorder and provide insight into how it shapes the lives of individuals, families, and communities.

Chapter 2

Searching for Answers

The Evolving Psychiatric View of Antisocial Personality Disorder

FEAR AND FASCINATION

As a youth, he fought with other boys, stabbed animals with red-hot irons, became a thief, and spent time in a juvenile detention center. He was an assassin by age 22, exiled to Syria and then Egypt before his return and rise to power in Iraq. Reported to have shot and killed a cabinet member during a meeting, he caused the deaths of thousands in gas attacks on Kurdistan, an eight-year conflict with Iran, the disastrous invasion of Kuwait, and the ensuing Persian Gulf War. According to biographers Efraim Karsh and Inari Rautsi, Saddam Hussein shared Adolph Hitler's "Darwinian world view in which only the fittest survive and where the end justifies the means. Both lacked the ability for personal empathy and possessed neither moral inhibitions nor respect for human life."[1] And, like Hitler, Saddam had an ignominious end, although at the end of a hangman's noose, rather than by a self-inflicted gunshot to the head.

The cloudy details of Hussein's life echo a connection traced by many writers of history and literature: Adults who defy social norms often establish a pattern of misbehavior in childhood, sometimes seeming to live without a conscience, to shirk the rules and expectations that keep most of us in check. They show a disturbing lack of empathy and fail to learn from their experiences, always blaming someone else for their problems and misdeeds. Such people can explain why the shopkeeper deserves to be robbed, why the spouse asks to be beaten, why their every betrayal is justified. Preoccupied with their own whims and desires, yet lacking any ability for introspection, these individuals do whatever is necessary to reach their ill-conceived goals. Rarely do they consider that they might be wrong.

In studying antisocial personality disorder (ASP), psychiatrists seek to answer a central question about the nature of bad behavior: Why do some individuals seem destined for lives of deception, violence, and harm to others? Why do they seem to lack a conscience? While men like Saddam Hussein may not meet every criterion for the psychiatric concept of ASP, their lives stand in undeniable contrast to the norm. These men fascinate us because they personify extremes of wickedness; but perhaps more subversive and certainly more widespread are the mundane ills that these men perpetrate, insults that gnaw at the fabric of society: petty crime, dishonesty and deception, the secret violence that happens inside families. All are commonly found in ASP.

The most recent edition of the American Psychiatric Association's *Diagnostic and Statistical Manual of Mental Disorders, Fourth Edition, Text Revision (DSM-IV-TR)*, a compendium of recognized psychiatric conditions, defines a personality disorder as "an enduring pattern of inner experience and behavior that deviates markedly from the expectations of the individual's culture, is pervasive and inflexible, has an onset in adolescence or early adulthood, is stable over time, and leads to distress or impairment."[2] *DSM-IV-TR* criteria for ASP require an established pattern of behaviors and attitudes that deny or violate the rights of others, including crime and other violations of social norms, deceit, impulsivity, aggression, recklessness, irresponsibility, and lack of remorse. Evidence of unusual childhood misbehavior—*conduct disorder* in current psychiatric parlance—must also be present. Only individuals who are older than 18 can be diagnosed with ASP, and psychiatrists must rule out other serious mental disorders like schizophrenia before making this diagnosis. Antisocial personality disorder symptoms and diagnostic criteria will be discussed more fully in the next chapter.

This chapter traces the history of ASP as a psychiatric disorder, from the first recorded case studies of antisocials to the development of contemporary standards for diagnosis and the discovery of correlations between ASP and gender, age, socioeconomic status, and other important risk factors. It also tells the story of Ernie, a man whose lifetime of antisocial behavior underscores the fact that ASP is a real and destructive psychiatric problem.

HISTORICAL BACKGROUND

In the early 19th century, Philippe Pinel, a founding father of psychiatry who unchained patients at the Bicêtre—a Paris hospital for insane men—and thus pioneered the humane treatment of the mentally ill, observed people subject to explosive and irrational violence, including one who hurled a woman down a well during a fit of rage.[3] Despite their behavior, such patients seemed to understand their actions and surroundings and did not display the bizarre delusions and frightening hallucinations associated with insanity. Pinel used the term *manie sans délire*—mania without delirium—to describe cases in which violent outbursts appeared unmotivated by an underlying psychiatric disturbance. His clinical vignettes became the first case studies of antisocial personality.

Although Pinel was struck by such behavior, he was at a loss to explain it. Benjamin Rush, a physician who signed the Declaration of Independence and founded the Pennsylvania Hospital, the first psychiatric facility in the United States, took Pinel's work a step further, describing habitual, deliberate bad behavior and positing a cause. In 1812, he wrote about one patient, the daughter of a prominent Philadelphian, who was "addicted to every kind of mischief. Her mischief and wickedness had no intervals while she was awake, except when she was kept busy in some steady and difficult employment." Rush theorized that such cases stemmed from a "defective organization in those parts of the body which are occupied by the moral faculties of the mind."[4] Although observing that the behavior was willful, he broke new ground with his suggestion, however vague, that it stemmed from a brain disorder. His work anticipated the results of neuroscience research that would come nearly two centuries later.

English physician James Prichard observed, like Rush, that some otherwise normal people engage in willful behavior that violates social norms and, in 1835, he coined a term to describe their state.

In his *Treatise on Insanity and Other Disorders Affecting the Mind*, he labeled it *moral insanity* and explained its difference from traditional notions of madness: "The intellectual faculties appear to have sustained little or no injury, while the disorder is manifested principally or alone in the state of the feelings, temper or habits. . . . In these cases the individual is found to be incapable ... of conducting himself with decency and propriety, having undergone a morbid change."[5] Prichard's use of the word *moral* predicted a significant facet of ASP as it is now understood. Many antisocials seem to have little moral sense, feeling no obligation to society or their peers and no respect for the regulations that most of us follow. Prichard's work also roused the medicalization argument that still rages today. His contemporaries worried that theorizing about diseases or defects of morality would result in diagnoses that could absolve individuals of responsibility for their actions, excusing them from punishment for social transgressions.

Although Prichard's concept of moral insanity helped shape how recurrent antisocial behavior was understood, the term itself did not stick. One that did, however, was introduced by German psychiatrists around 1890. Julius Koch, a leader of the group, coined the term "psychopathic inferiority," and used it to describe a broad range of deviant behaviors and eccentricities that implied the disorder was constitutional or inbred, further solidifying the notion that for some, antisocial behavior is a way of life.

The word *psychopathic* was popularized decades later, largely by two authors working independently. Scottish psychiatrist David Henderson published the book *Psychopathic States* in 1939, defining three types of psychopaths.[6] The *predominantly inadequate psychopath*, according to Henderson, siphons a living off society by swindling or pilfering, crimes that involve little overt aggression. Vagrants and petty thieves fall into this category. The *predominantly aggressive psychopath* is a potentially dangerous individual subject to

fits of violence. *Creative psychopaths* are highly individualistic, sometimes eccentric people determined to "carve out a way for themselves
irrespective of the obstacles which bestow their path," including,
in Henderson's view, such prominent and respected figures as Joan
of Arc and Lawrence of Arabia. (Many traits ascribed to this group
today define *narcissistic personality disorder*, which is characterized by
extreme self-centeredness.) We see in these categories, especially the
inadequates and the aggressives, the types of patients who today are
regarded as antisocial.

Henderson's American contemporary, psychiatrist Hervey
Cleckley, was far more influential in the United States, developing
perhaps the first coherent description of antisocial personality in his
now-classic *The Mask of Sanity—An Attempt to Clarify Some Issues
About the So-Called Psychopathic Personality.*[7] Revised four times after
its initial publication in 1941, the book remains worthwhile reading for its fascinating case studies and the author's uncompromising
opinions. Although Cleckley is better known for *The Three Faces of
Eve*, the story of a woman with many strikingly different personalities, co-authored with Corbett H. Thigpen, *The Mask of Sanity* documents his true legacy.

Cleckley defined the condition, in terms similar to contemporary
views of ASP, as a disorder distinct from other psychiatric problems
and behavioral abnormalities. Through a series of case vignettes, he
showed how the disorder transcends social class and argued that
psychopaths exhibit an extraordinary lack of depression or anxiety. According to Cleckley, a constellation of 16 traits define the
psychopath:

- Superficial charm and "good" intelligence
- Absence of delusions and other signs of irrational thinking
- Absence of "nervousness" or other signs of psychoneurotic
  disturbances

- Unreliability
- Untruthfulness and insincerity
- Lack of remorse or shame
- Inadequately motivated antisocial behavior
- Poor judgment and failure to learn from experience
- Pathological egocentricity and incapacity for love
- General poverty in major affective reactions
- Specific loss of insight
- Unresponsiveness in general interpersonal relations
- Fantastic and uninviting behavior with drinking and sometimes without
- Suicide rarely carried out
- Sex life impersonal, trivial, and poorly integrated
- Failure to follow any life plan

Cleckley wrestled with the question of responsibility raised during Prichard's time, arguing that the disorder he described should never be considered an excuse for misbehavior. He realized that brutal acts of violence like rape and murder might be explained away as evidence of a serious mental disorder, to be treated as illness rather than crime. Psychopaths, he argued, are not insane. They know right from wrong and are not out of touch with reality; their acts, however deplorable, are deliberate and purposeful. Cleckley insisted that good lawyers invariably compound the problems of psychopathic clients by helping them escape responsibility for their crimes.

For Cleckley, the psychopath was the "forgotten man of psychiatry [who] probably causes more unhappiness and more perplexity to the public than all other mentally disordered patients combined."[8] The psychopath's condition was ignored not only by society at large, he complained, but also by psychiatrists, whose texts paid it little attention. He feared medical students would conclude that the "psychopath is an unimportant figure, probably seldom encountered in psychiatric practice."[9]

Cleckley's ideas, along with Henderson's, were incorporated into the first *Diagnostic and Statistical Manual of Mental Disorders* (*DSM-I*), published in 1952. *DSM-I* was the first formal effort by the American Psychiatric Association to catalogue in one volume the different disorders encountered in the expanding field of psychiatry. Chronic antisocial acts and attitudes were classified as subtypes of *sociopathic personality disturbance,* one of several personality disorders listed. The subtype *antisocial reaction* was applied to individuals "who are always in trouble, profiting neither from experience nor punishment, and maintaining no real loyalties to any person, group, or code. They are frequently callous and hedonistic, showing marked emotional immaturity, with lack of sense of responsibility, lack of judgment, and an ability to rationalize their behavior so that it appears warranted, reasonable, and justified."[10] The *dyssocial reaction* referred to those who "manifest disregard for the usual social codes, and often come into conflict with them." These individuals often adhere to the values and codes of their "own predatory, criminal, or other social group." Other subtypes involved sexual deviance and addiction to drugs or alcohol.

One of my study subjects, Ernie, came of age as psychiatry was constructing the terms that would define his condition. His story is a sadly familiar tale of youthful misbehavior, crime, addiction, and assorted other problems—a pattern of trouble seen repeatedly in patients with ASP. Like all antisocials, Ernie chose his path early in life. Or perhaps his path chose him.

ERNIE'S STORY: 1958

The physicians who evaluated Ernie in 1958 had probably read their Cleckley and *DSM-I.* Before them was a young man who had, by all accounts, lived a life of trouble: fights with other boys, expulsion from school, petty theft, a two-year stint in the reformatory by age 18. Admitting Ernie to the University of Iowa Psychopathic Hospital, a young psychiatrist-in-training reviewed the boy's records and surmised that Ernie had a "sociopathic personality disturbance, antisocial type," adding a hopeful note that brief hospitalization might help him. An older, experienced clinician was less sanguine, describing the patient as "replete with surface phenomenon [sic] of lack of guilt and anxiety in a self-centered, uncontrolled person." He had seen it all before, too many times.

Ernie had entered the hospital voluntarily and with the support of his adoptive parents, John and Dorothy Walker. They had met the boy 10 years earlier, welcoming him into their home as the child they could never conceive. Ernie came to them with an IQ of 112, a love of sports, and an engaging smile, so charming that the Walkers paid little attention to the behavior problems glossed over by officials at the adoption agency, who had blamed the boy's troubles on an unstable living situation. A good home would surely straighten him out, and the Walkers offered just that—a tidy house filled with toys and clothes and overlooking a large yard in a fine neighborhood. But, as they discovered, Ernie's problems were much more than they could ever expect to cure.

The Walkers thought that Ernie's troubles stemmed from some unresolved trauma, maybe anger at them or at his biological parents. Perhaps Ernie himself believed it too. He told the doctors at the hospital that his tendency to act out frightened him, that he wasn't sure he could keep himself in line. He didn't want to end up in prison. Over a period of days, physicians, nurses, and social workers slowly peeled back the layers of Ernie's history, comparing it to information from the Walkers and the boy's records. They hoped to uncover anything that would reveal a cause for his misbehavior or at least enable them to give his problem a name.

The interviewers described Ernie as an attractive lad preoccupied by his fashionable "duck tail" hairstyle: "He is obviously quite proud of his [hair] and brushes his hands lovingly over it." The boy smoked as he told his story, flicking ashes onto the linoleum while stoically recounting his abuse, misery, and abandonment. His natural father was a factory man and an alcoholic, quick to lay a hand on a rambunctious child. Ernie's mother was this man's fifth wife, "screwier than hell," as Ernie described her. He was six years old when his father walked out, leaving Ernie and his two brothers to their mentally ill mother, who soon gave them up to the state. That was the last Ernie had seen of her, but he didn't seem to mind. After all, he noted, she had abandoned him and thus dissolved their bond. Foster care meant being separated from his brothers and bounced from home to home until the Walkers came along. As Ernie told it, they were tyrants hiding behind a polished façade: Dot beat him with a whip when he violated her strict demands for punctuality, cleanliness, and decorum; John was stern and cold. Their home, although stocked with wonderful things, was an emotional void by Ernie's sensational account.

Among his earliest memories were stealing from candy stores, slipping cash from his father's wallet, and, after he was adopted by the Walkers, pocketing toys from the comfortable homes of playmates. He was smart, but his low grades and misdeeds brought strong reprimands from teachers and time spent standing in the corner or staying after school. His true calling was crime, and soon he was shoplifting clothing and records, burglarizing churches, and hot-wiring cars. In high school, he was caught robbing a fellow student and was sent by his harried parents to an expensive military academy, which soon kicked him out. At age 16, he was found stealing purses from a bowling alley and was confined to a boys' reformatory.

There he discovered, by his own account, a nightmarish hole of Dickensian proportions. A skeptical interviewer wrote that Ernie "gave a rambling account of solitary confinement, cutting [his] hair, shoveling coal, etc." In fact, Ernie had earned his time in solitary by slashing another boy with a razor blade, an event he refused to discuss. He seemed proud of his success at manipulating the reformatory staff, bragging of how he had bought beer and wine by paying off the right people with a generous allowance from the Walkers. Although he had no history of drug use, Ernie described considerable drinking. He also boasted of losing his virginity at 15 and having sex with numerous girls in the two months since his reformatory stay ended (a "rather lurid account," wrote one of the doctors). Although his interviewers attributed his sexual history to adolescent exaggeration, they noted that, at the time of his admission, he was living with a woman he met on the midway of the Iowa State Fair a month earlier.

The psychiatrists found no evidence of depression, delusions, or hallucinations, and wrote: "He is well oriented and performs well on tests of intellectual function." A physical examination was unremarkable, and an electroencephalographic tracing was normal, ruling out organic brain injury. Although they managed to complete their assessment and begin treatment, neither the doctors nor the Walkers could persuade Ernie to stay at the hospital. He showed no interest in psychotherapy, sat bored through group sessions, and insulted the staff. After 15 days, he announced that he was leaving to see his girlfriend, and the doctors described him as unimproved upon discharge. The final diagnosis remained "sociopathic personality disturbance, antisocial type."

THE BIRTH OF THE ANTISOCIAL

Ernie had become a sociopath, in the jargon of the day, based on his records and self-described history, but also on the impressions of his physicians. The ability to assess and interpret behavior is an important component of psychiatry, but the basis for diagnosis has changed since Ernie's hospitalization in the 1950s. Since then, a concerted effort has been made to solidify the criteria used to diagnose mental disorders. For personality disorders like ASP, these advances have been substantial.

The term *antisocial personality disorder* was introduced in 1968, with the second edition of the *DSM*, which gave the condition an identity separate from the addictions and deviant sexuality. Like *sociopath*, the word *antisocial* refers to a reaction against society and a rejection of its rules and obligations. *DSM-II* described the term as "reserved for individuals who are basically unsocialized and whose behavior pattern brings them repeatedly into conflict with society. They are incapable of significant loyalty to individuals, groups or social values. They are grossly selfish, callous, irresponsible, impulsive, and unable to feel guilt or to learn from experience and punishment. Frustration tolerance is low. They tend to blame others or offer plausible rationalizations for their behavior. A mere history of repeated legal or social offenses is not sufficient to justify this diagnosis."[11] The dyssocial subtype of *DSM-I* was relegated to a category of "conditions without manifest psychiatric disorder," reserved for those who were considered psychiatrically normal but who followed criminal pursuits, such as racketeers and prostitutes.

Although the term *antisocial personality disorder* has achieved wide acceptance among psychiatrists, it was more than a decade before diagnostic criteria for the disorder were set forth in *DSM-III*, published in 1980. The third *DSM* replaced the vague and imprecise descriptions of *DSM-II* with lists of specific criteria that must be met to justify any psychiatric diagnosis. The criteria are fully discussed in the following chapter.

In developing the criteria for *DSM-III*, Columbia University psychiatrist Robert Spitzer, and others charged with shepherding the process, were greatly influenced by the work of sociologist Lee Robins and her colleagues at Washington University in St. Louis.[12] In her seminal book *Deviant Children Grown Up*, published in 1966, Robins detailed specific behavioral symptoms that became the basis for the ASP criteria in *DSM-III*, such as inability to maintain consistent employment, illegal and aggressive behavior, and sexual promiscuity.[13] Although *The Mask of* Sanity was well-known, Cleckley's work in defining psychopathy was thought to include psychological traits that would not easily lend themselves to reliable assessment by psychiatrists. For example, superficial charm, callousness, untruthfulness and insincerity, and lack of guilt or shame require subjective judgments about character. Spitzer and his committee preferred the behavioral criteria used by Robins, believing them more likely to result in reliable diagnoses.[14] Her work also showed that these criteria identified a well-defined group of significantly troubled individuals with shared symptoms and prognosis. In short, the criteria were reliable *and* valid, terms indicating that different psychiatrists could agree on the diagnosis with a high degree of confidence, but also confirming that the diagnosis was clinically meaningful.

From the beginning, the goal of the *DSM* was to standardize psychiatric classification and language as a basis for research and practice, promoting communication among psychiatrists and other mental health professionals. Nevertheless, the publication of *DSM-III* riled many psychiatrists. Some complained that the diagnostic criteria were arbitrary or reduced the art of diagnosis to a numbers game by mandating that patients meet a specified number of criteria for a given disorder. Certainly, the new approach stripped some of the mystery from psychiatry and helped reshape the fuzzy and impressionistic way that psychiatrists were thought to practice their craft. Diagnostic criteria improved communication, provided a simpler approach to psychiatric assessment, and made diagnoses more reliable. This meant that psychiatrists in different parts of the country, or indeed different parts of the world, when seeing the same symptoms in their patients, would arrive at the same diagnosis. Pioneered by psychiatrists, such standards now are becoming popular in other medical specialties.

DSM-III was also criticized from outside the mental health professions. To some, its attempt to define hundreds of disorders sliced psychiatry too thin, proposing a pathology for every imaginable brand of aberrant behavior. The most cynical complaints portrayed the *DSM* as a money grab by psychiatrists, an ever-expanding catalog of ostensibly treatable disorders for which mental health professionals could charge their patients. In truth, *DSM-III* and its successors are part of the ongoing effort to separate real mental health problems from normal feelings and behaviors, and to ensure professional communication and conformity. For example, the diagnostic criteria that define ASP offer a framework to distinguish it from ordinary instances of misbehavior. They provide a more stable and consistent ground for diagnosis than previous descriptions of the disorder.

The ASP criteria were simplified in later editions of the *DSM*, including a minor revision in 1987 (*DSM-III-R*), and a fourth edition in 1994 (*DSM-IV*). In 2000, a text revision was published, but there were no additional changes to the criteria (*DSM-IV-TR*).[15] Motivated by concerns that psychological characteristics important to ASP were excluded in the definition, lack of remorse was added as a criterion in *DSM-IV*.

The *DSM* story continues, and a fifth edition (*DSM-5*) is scheduled for release in May 2013, but there will be no changes to the ASP criteria. (One notable change was that its authors chose to use the Arabic numeral "5" rather than a Roman numeral!) Although there may be some changes in the criteria, ASP will to continue as one of the acknowledged personality disorders. Publication is expected in 2013.

A CONNECTION WITH PSYCHOPATHY

Cleckley's approach to psychopathy in *The Mask of Sanity* greatly influenced the thinking of many psychiatrists and psychologists, some of whom who were dissatisfied by the decision to focus on observable behaviors in *DSM-III* at the expense of important psychological motives or interpersonal aspects thought to underlie antisocial behavior. In the wake of these concerns, interest developed in defining and researching *psychopathy*, as an entity distinct from ASP, defined by symptoms such as glibness, callousness, lack of emotional connection to others, and having an incapacity for guilt or remorse.

Robert Hare, a psychologist at the University of British Columbia, has been one of the leading champions of recognizing psychopathy as a clinical disorder. He developed what has become the main tool for identifying psychopathy, publishing the first version in 1980. Now known as the Psychopathy Checklist–Revised (PCL-R), the questionnaire is given by trained individuals to assess the disorder as he and others have defined it. Much of his work, described in *Without Conscience—The Disturbing World of the Psychopaths Among Us*, has taken place in prison settings, where the checklist has proven useful in identifying people with psychopathic traits, as well as in predicting recidivism (reoffending) and parole violations.[16] Hare has a wide following, and psychopathy has gained ground as a topic of investigation, perhaps because it is both measurable (using the PCL-R) and easier for many to grasp as a clinical disorder than is ASP. For that reason, many of the research studies referred to throughout this book concern psychopaths, not antisocials. Wherever possible, I note the distinction.

Nevertheless, psychopathy is *not* included in *DSM-IV-TR*, nor will it be included in *DSM-5*. For that reason, it is not the subject of this book, as my goal is to focus on ASP because it is the officially recognized disorder. The two conditions overlap, and Hare has himself noted that most antisocial persons are not psychopaths, as defined by his checklist, although nearly *all* psychopaths meet criteria for ASP. Estimates are that about a third of incarcerated men with ASP are psychopaths.[17] My own view, and that of others, is that psychopathy lies along a continuum of severity with ASP and likely constitutes its most severe variant.[18]

ERNIE'S STORY: 1988

Tracking down Ernie 30 years after his hospitalization was not easy, but just as my research team thought we had reached a dead end, one of his relatives called to say he was living in a small Iowa town. Cathy Butler, my research assistant at the time, found his alias in the phone book and reached him at home. He listened to her explain the study and agreed to an interview. A week later, Cathy made the 90-minute drive to meet him and found his street in a decaying neighborhood. Two men on a corner glanced up as she passed, suspending and then resuming what looked to Cathy like a drug deal. Ernie's house was a worn structure sagging over a ragged yard and covered with flaking yellow paint. Faded pink bed sheets were draped across a large front window, and a pair of scrawny cats skulked into hiding as Cathy stepped from the car. She mustered her nerve and approached the front door, giving it a firm knock. No one responded. After a few tries, she returned to the car, disappointed at being stood up. When she called Ernie later, he claimed he had forgotten the interview while on an alcoholic binge. They arranged another meeting.

Ernie, now 48, looked much older than his age, and Cathy's nursing background told her that he appeared chronically ill, shaking with what may have been alcohol withdrawal. Bald but for a fringe of dirty hair, he wore a filthy overcoat and had several days' growth of beard and a mouthful of stained teeth. His house was dark, stank of urine and mildew, and was nearly as cold as the gray November day outside. Ernie explained that the chill air was due to a broken furnace. He fumbled for a cigarette and lit up while Cathy again described the nature of the study. When he began to speak, she thought of the duck-tailed boy in the hospital, smoking and telling his story.

He had been incarcerated after all, spending 17 years in the state penitentiary, an experience that he said still haunted his dreams. Small spaces reminded him of solitary confinement, and the murders he witnessed—plus one he claimed to have committed—came back to him sometimes. Soon after being jailed, he had managed an escape. Although he was captured and returned after two months, the details of the escape story made it all the more bizarre. He had been helped by his biological mother, and the incident marked the beginning of a sexual relationship between them. Despite the unexpected admission, Cathy remained cool, asking if the experience had caused him any problems. He offered that it might have "mixed up" his feelings about women, then added, "I'll never get over it." When he said nothing more, Cathy moved on.

Armed robbery, receiving stolen goods, using aliases, burglary, drunk driving, and attempted murder appeared on his record of more than 20 arrests. He had been in mental hospitals at least nine times; all of the admissions, he claimed, were alcohol-related. In addition to his lasting alcohol habit, he had used marijuana, amphetamines, cocaine, tranquilizers, and heroin.

He shared the three-bedroom home with six others, including his four children—ages 4 to 11—his common-law wife, and a 15-year-old stepson. The wife, stepson, and oldest child earned the family's living, supplemented by illegal welfare payments and Food Stamps. Although Ernie claimed to paint cars occasionally in his garage, he admitted a recent lack of work. His wife cleaned houses, his stepson flipped burgers, and his son carried newspapers, but Ernie himself had never held a full-time job or maintained part-time work for longer than 60 days. He estimated having held almost 150 jobs during the previous decade. He and his wife had met in a mental hospital some five years earlier, and Ernie noted that she took unidentified tranquilizers for an unnamed illness. The relationship was a bad one, fraught with constant fights that occasionally ended with the police at their door. When drunk, Ernie sometimes beat his wife and the children, but felt powerless to do much about it. "They're used to it by now," he remarked.

Ernie grinned when Cathy mentioned how difficult he had been to find. "I just like to move," he said, tracing his life in six states under many different names. Cathy suspected that his more than 20 moves had been motivated by a need to escape—from rental payments, creditors, or the police. When asked about the Walkers, he offered tearful regrets for losing contact once they had severed their relationship with him. He had no acquaintances outside his family and never socialized, except for trips to bars and occasional Alcoholics Anonymous meetings at a nearby church.

He hadn't settled down, he said, and still lived a reckless life, spending his little money heedlessly and getting into frequent fights. Weeks earlier, he had been arrested on public intoxication and assault charges. He understood that his behavior violated most social norms, but he didn't seem to care. In fact, he said, he "still got a charge out of doing dangerous things."

"Like what?" Cathy asked.

"You don't really want to know," he answered, lips curled in a teasing smile.

With that, Cathy ended the interview.

LINKS TO ANTISOCIAL PERSONALITY DISORDER

By providing more precise criteria to define ASP, the *DSM* has made it easier to identify, bringing greater consistency to the diagnosis and setting a foundation for research that continues to advance our understanding of the disorder. Using the contemporary definition of ASP, a number of studies have shown that it is more likely to be found among certain groups, including men and people living in poverty, even while it crosses cultural, racial, and other boundaries. These findings offer psychiatrists and other mental health professionals additional clues with which to pursue the disorder, both in working with patients and in carrying out research.

The most significant epidemiologic feature of ASP is that it is almost exclusively a disorder of men. Depending on the population surveyed, ASP affects from two to eight times more men than women. One explanation for this disparity comes from researchers partial to genetic explanations: Men with a particular gene or set of genes might be predisposed toward ASP, whereas women who carry it might instead develop another condition, for instance *somatization disorder*, which is characterized by multiple unexplained physical symptoms. Other researchers attribute gender differences in ASP to cultural norms: Women learn to turn anger inward, while men learn to express it in outward actions. Because overt aggression is less likely to be tolerated in women, perhaps they act out in less obvious ways.[19] This could mean that the perceived gender difference is largely artificial, that women are as likely as men to be antisocial but go undiagnosed. Further discussion about women and ASP is found in Chapter 3.

Antisocial personality disorder also has been linked with both poverty and homelessness, although it occurs as well among people whose socioeconomic standing muffles its expression.[20] The connection is not surprising, considering the antisocial lifestyle. Poor school achievement, inconsistent work histories, and irresponsible behavior lead to low-wage, dead-end jobs with little hope for advancement, or to intermittent or chronic unemployment. Poverty and homelessness create situations in which antisocial impulses are more likely to be acted upon and observed. For some, crime becomes a means of survival, while others come to rely on public or private largesse. Antisocials rarely overcome years of lost educational and career opportunities to catch up economically with their non-antisocial peers. The possibility that economic disadvantage also may contribute to the development of ASP—making poverty a cause of the disorder as well as a symptom—will be taken up in Chapter 6.

Other circumstances also show especially high rates of the disorder, further reflecting the drift of antisocials toward certain problems and outcomes. Research suggests that up to 80% of men and 65% of women in American prisons meet the criteria for ASP, but these extraordinarily high figures may overstate the prevalence.[21] More recent data suggest that the percentage of inmates with ASP has dropped, perhaps because harsh drug sentencing laws lead to the incarceration of otherwise normal people who get caught up in the drug trade.[22] Nonetheless, the disorder is clearly much more common behind bars than in the general public—hardly surprising, since criminal behavior is a main facet of ASP.

Yet crime is only one aspect of ASP, and not all criminals are antisocial. Some lack the history of childhood misbehavior that helps define ASP. Others commit isolated crimes of passion or opportunity, or repeatedly carry out specific types of crimes without showing the broad spectrum of misbehavior that characterizes ASP. Explaining all offenses as the product of ASP or lumping all violators together and calling crime itself a clinical disorder—a strategy adopted by Adrian Raine, a University of Pennsylvania psychologist—oversimplifies the roots of crime.[23] Nonetheless, ASP is undoubtedly a factor in many crimes, and the typical antisocial spends some time behind bars.

Antisocial personality disorder is also more common among patients seen in psychiatric hospitals and clinics, although ASP is seldom the problem that motivates them to seek treatment. Antisocial patients in these settings are typically seen for depression, substance abuse, suicidal behavior, or interpersonal and marital problems, with their underlying ASP frequently overlooked or ignored. Among some patient groups, ASP rates are extremely high. Up to half of those in treatment for alcoholism meet criteria for the disorder, and the rates are even higher among heroin and other drug addicts.[24] This increased prevalence of ASP among patients is not confined to mental health or substance abuse programs. One study found that 8% of men and 3% of women seen by 64 primary care physicians—internists, family physicians, and other generalists who treat most common health problems—met *DSM* criteria for the disorder.[25] The lesson here is that the disorder is common and is highly likely to show up in just about any medical setting.

Both ASP and antisocial behavior in general are more common among young people. Just as most persons arrested and incarcerated are younger than 30, the Epidemiologic Catchment Area (ECA) study shows the highest concentration of ASP in people aged 25–44, and that rates of the disorder diminish with advancing age.[26] Because ASP is considered lifelong, we might expect prevalence—the number of affected persons—to increase with age, yet the opposite occurs: The diagnosis is *less* likely in older groups of people. There are several possible explanations. Some individuals may be unable to recall their youthful indiscretions, while more than a few simply lie about their past. Others improve to the point at which they no longer meet the diagnostic criteria. Some continue to exhibit symptoms but attract relatively little attention. This is what psychiatrist Julio Arboleda-Florez and psychologist Heather Holley found when they examined the arrest records of 38 antisocial men aged 41–67 years. Criminal convictions declined after age 27, even though one-third of the subjects remained criminally active throughout adulthood.[27] Last, because many antisocials die prematurely from suicide, murder, or reckless accidents, they are not around for late-life surveys.

One characteristic with scant relationship to ASP is ethnicity. This may come as a surprise to some, because of the disorder's high prevalence in low-income urban communities and prisons, settings where racial and ethnic minorities are overrepresented. In the ECA study, rates of the disorder among Americans of European, African, and Hispanic ancestry showed little variation in prevalence across ethnic groups.[28] Close examination of ECA data reveals some racial differences among those reporting ASP symptoms. African American antisocials more commonly reported a history of violent behavior and arrests, whereas whites typically admitted nonviolent symptoms, such as troubled work histories, vagrancy, and minor criminal offenses. Bottom line: For most, ASP is an equal opportunity disorder for people of all races, its expression shaped by one's social environment, which perhaps accounts for the few differences observed among the groups.

A TYPICAL ANTISOCIAL

I wish I could say Ernie's case is rare, but stories like his are sadly common among men diagnosed as antisocial. Having spent years in prison, drifted from place to place and job to job, become mired in alcoholism and poverty, Ernie settled for a life bereft of opportunity and advancement, or indeed happiness. Although he had grown old—years before his time—little about him had changed aside from the fact that he had given up felonies, at least for the moment. Based on the events of his life, even considering his gift for hyperbole, Ernie was as antisocial at follow-up as he had been in 1958. The cocksure young man with the duck tail and attitude was gone, except for a few boastful lies. But the old man who replaced him showed no remorse. His dismal outcome was not a surprise, for ASP seldom remits, its many symptoms continuing to take their toll throughout the lives of most antisocials.

Chapter 3

Bad Boys to Bad Men

The Symptoms of
Antisocial Personality Disorder

OFF THE WAGON

Edward Honneker looked bored as he sprawled in a stiff wooden chair, casting occasional glances out the window and calmly answering the psychiatrist's questions. Asked why he had been sent to the hospital, Ed smirked and skirted responsibility for the actions that had put him there. "Well, it's happened before," he said. "You see, I'm one of those guys who starts out good but falls off the wagon eventually."

In truth, Ed had started out badly and stayed on that course. The son of a prominent Midwestern judge, he had a reputation for emotional instability and other troubles that began during childhood. In elementary school, he lied to teachers, cheated on exams, and battled other boys during recess. His behavior grew worse as he advanced through the grades, until he was expelled from junior high school. The public schools refused to take him back, so Ed's embarrassed parents packed him off to a military academy in a nearby state, where he adapted to the rigid discipline and successfully earned a high school diploma in 1942.

The Second World War raged in Europe and the Pacific, but Ed was assigned a stateside post when he joined the Army, much to his parents' relief. Again, he managed to do fairly well in the structured military environment and eventually received an honorable discharge, despite experiencing an episode of depression that led to his first psychiatric hospitalization. In 1946, he left the service and set out for California, hoping to find an exciting life far from home. After waiting tables for a while, he lived off monthly checks from his parents, preferring to spend his time lazing on the beach, playing pool, or getting drunk. On one of those carefree days, he married a young woman who left him several months later, disappointed by his shiftlessness and lack of drive. After she gave birth to their baby girl, Ed refused to give any parental or financial support.

Blaming the stress and expense of his divorce, Ed began writing bad checks and had his first brush with the law, a conviction that landed him a three-month jail term plus probation. Having tasted punishment, he returned home to Iowa at his parents' urging. But only two months passed before he was arrested again, this time for using false checks to stage a shopping spree that included a new Buick, which was to be his ticket back to California. He was barely across the state line when the police caught up with him and returned him home in deep trouble. Once again, his father was there to bail him out, using his considerable influence to have the charges dropped and pressuring his son to enroll at the University of Iowa. A third check-kiting charge in 1950 put Ed before a judge, who demanded he receive psychiatric evaluation.

Ed's father accompanied him to the hospital and explained to the doctors that Ed had always been unstable, never engaging in any gainful activity. Although he cared about his boy, he was tired of rescuing him from his mistakes and was shamed by his son's actions. Hoping the psychiatrists could find a reason and remedy for his son's persistent troubles, he described Ed as an expert manipulator who was "always maneuvering himself into various positions." By the time Ed left the hospital days later, his doctors had made a diagnosis, but Ed never gave them a chance to help. Instead, he returned to the road, writing a bad check here, crafting an elaborate con there, always remaining beyond the grasp of his family and others who sought to help him.

Ed's childhood behavior problems and failures at school recall Ernie's. Both men grew up showing many of the signs that characterize young antisocials and that bloomed into full-fledged antisocial personality disorder (ASP) symptoms by adulthood. At age 5, the antisocial child bites and hits other youngsters; at 10, he skips school and shoplifts; by 16, he sells drugs or steals cars; at 22, his crimes escalate to robbery or rape; at age 30, he beats his wife and children; and, by 45, he drinks too much and cheats his employer. Although the cycle of misbehavior shifts with changes in circumstances, it remains a force throughout the person's life. The symptoms of ASP vary, but the similarities among cases are often more remarkable than are the differences.

GROWING UP ANTISOCIAL

Many of us tend to idealize childhood as a magical time unburdened by the demands of adult life, often forgetting its pains and its sometimes unpleasant lessons. Even in childhood, there are set expectations that most children quickly learn and obey. Every child misbehaves now and then, and normal developmental stages like the "terrible twos" are noted for characteristic rebelliousness. But when bad behavior is persistent, repetitive, and wide-ranging, a diagnosis of *conduct disorder* may be fitting. The American Psychiatric Association's *Diagnostic and Statistical Manual of Mental Disorders, Fourth Edition, Text Revision* (*DSM-IV-TR*) requires that adults diagnosed with ASP have a history of conduct disorder, even though it may have gone unrecognized at the time.

Conduct disorder is defined in the *DSM-IV-TR* as a pattern of behavior in which the basic rights of others or major age-appropriate rules or social norms are repeatedly violated.[1] Like ASP, conduct disorder occurs mainly in boys, many of whom are also diagnosed with attention-deficit/hyperactivity disorder (ADHD). Evident even at a very young age, conduct disorder affects from 5% to 15% of all children.[2] Critics of the conduct disorder diagnosis raise some of the same concerns voiced about ASP, warning that it medicalizes bad behavior. Some argue that it has the unintended consequence of excusing children from responsibility for their actions, permitting parents to blame bad behavior

THE DSM-IV-TR CRITERIA FOR CONDUCT DISORDER ARE:

A. A repetitive and persistent pattern of behavior in which the basic rights of others or major age-appropriate societal norms or rules are violated, as manifested by the presence of three (or more) of the following criteria in the past 12 months, with at least one criterion present in the past 6 months.

Aggression to People and Animals
1. Often bullies, threatens, or intimidates others
2. Often initiates physical fights
3. Has used a weapon that can cause serious physical harm to others (e.g., a bat, brick, broken bottle, knife, gun)
4. Has been physically cruel to people
5. Has been physically cruel to animals
6. Has stolen while confronting a victim (e.g., mugging, purse snatching, extortion, armed robbery)
7. Has forced someone into sexual activity

Destruction of Property
8. Has deliberately engaged in fire setting with the intention of causing serious damage
9. Has deliberately destroyed others' property (other than by fire setting)

Deceitfulness or Theft
10. Has broken into someone else's house, building, or car
11. Often lies to obtain goods or favors or to avoid obligations (i.e., "cons" others)

(continued from previous page)

12. Has stolen items of nontrivial value without confronting a victim (e.g., shoplifting, but without breaking and entering; forgery)

Serious Violations of Rules

13. Often stays out at night despite parental prohibitions, beginning before age 13 years
14. Has run away from home overnight at least twice while living in parental or parental surrogate home (or once without returning for a lengthy period)
15. Often truant from school, beginning before age 13 years

B. The disturbance in behavior causes clinically significant impairment in social, academic, or occupational functioning.

C. If the individual is age 18 years or older, criteria are not met for antisocial personality disorder.

(Reprinted with permission from the *Diagnostic and Statistical Manual of Mental Disorders*, 4th ed. Text Revision. Copyright 2000, American Psychiatric Association.)

on the disorder rather than the child, or that it may label children for life with a stigmatizing diagnosis. Although the diagnosis must be used judiciously, it has legitimate value. By helping parents and mental health professionals recognize children with truly unusual histories of misbehavior, a conduct disorder diagnosis may inform decisions about how to raise and care for the child it affects.

In considering the diagnosis, mental health professionals look for misbehavior in four main areas: aggression toward people or animals, destruction of property, deceitfulness or theft, and serious violations of rules. A child with conduct disorder must meet at least 3 of 15 criteria divided among these four problem areas. These behavior problems must significantly impair the child's social, academic, or occupational functioning. In many ways, they resemble the symptoms of adult ASP.

DISPLAYING AGGRESSION

Aggression in children is a frequent subject of contemporary concern, as the media describe violent behavior once considered unthinkable among kids who seem to get younger with each passing report. In 1994, the *New York Times, Time* magazine, and other national publications told the story of a scrawny 11-year-old Chicago boy called "Yummy" for his love of cookies and Snickers bars. Murdered by his own street gang after allegedly killing a 14-year-old girl by mistake, Yummy's criminal record and reputation belied his youth. Neglected and abused, bounced from group homes to juvenile detention facilities, Yummy had used fire, knives, and guns to intimidate neighbors and other kids. In the few short years before his death, he was connected with at least 20 felonies, including drug possession and armed robbery. A psychiatric evaluation described him as impulsive and unpredictable, but one observer, quoted in *Time*, said the boy's future was all too easy to foretell: "What you've got here is a kid who was made and turned into a sociopath by the time he was three years old."[3] Yummy died at the hands of two brothers, aged 14 and 15, shot execution-style.

Violence is a common thread running through the lives of such children. In New York, a 13-year-old boy made national news by killing a four-year-old whom he savagely beat and sodomized with a stick. An ABC news profile detailed the young killer's history of behavior problems, beginning with head banging and temper tantrums, fascination with fire, and cruelty to animals.[4] The boy was tried as an adult, and his attorney argued that "A kid who would do this probably has something very wrong with his brain." But like most children with serious conduct problems, the boy showed no evidence of brain damage.

Although stories like these end in shocking acts of violence, many begin with patterns of aggressive behavior that define conduct disorder, patterns eventually taken to extremes. Of course, most childhood aggression, whether name-calling, shoving, or minor scuffles, is relatively benign and not the type of behavior that generates headlines or creates grave concerns. Bullies—the familiar characters who haunt school hallways and playgrounds—epitomize the aggressive tendencies found in some children.[5] They tend to come from environments where adult supervision is minimal and physical discipline teaches that "might makes right." Research shows that men who were bullies in childhood are more likely to commit criminal acts as adults and to engage in domestic violence—not surprising when one takes into account the link between conduct problems in childhood and ASP later in life.[6] However, not all schoolyard bullies are destined to become antisocial, and some learn to abandon their aggressive behavior.

But for others, mostly boys, fist fights, intimidation, and milder acts of aggression escalate to dangerous heights. These children gradually take up weapons in their fights—sometimes progressing to guns—and their crimes may increasingly involve physical intimidation or assault. Cruelty to animals is another form of childhood aggression linked with adult violence.[7] Many antisocial adults and children with conduct disorder have histories of abusing, torturing, or killing pets. Children who become antisocial as adults often are sexually active before their peers, engaging in early masturbation and sex play, sometimes forcing others to perform sexual acts. In some cases, childhood sexual activity is motivated by abuse from adults, abuse that is then reenacted on other children.[8]

DAMAGING PROPERTY

Destruction of property, ranging from petty vandalism to deadly games like starting fires, is symptomatic of conduct disorder. There is a difference between ordinary children who engage in occasional mischief and those who repeatedly hurl rocks through windows, kick over cemetery headstones, and go on destructive rampages. Their actions can bring major property damage or even death. Starting fires, like animal cruelty, is an especially alarming behavior that correlates highly with adult violence. In 1997, Betty Shabazz, widow of African American leader Malcolm X, died from injuries suffered in a fire set by her 12-year-old grandson, a boy said to have had behavior problems and a long-time fascination with flames.[9] A study of 36 murderers found that 58% set fires as children and 52% set fires as adolescents. Serial killer David Berkowitz, better known as the "Son of Sam," was reported to have started more than 1,400 fires in his youth.[10]

LYING AND STEALING

Children with conduct disorder learn how to evade responsibility for their misdeeds, and deceitfulness is the third major feature of the diagnosis. Lying comes naturally to these children, whose small fibs often grow into fanciful stories and blatant falsehoods. Some children become adept at telling complex lies to parents, teachers, and others, using deceit to cover up bad behavior or to gain rewards. Theft, or stealing without confrontation, is also common in conduct disorder, and may involve shoplifting or breaking into cars, homes, and businesses—crimes in which antisocial offenders like Tom, Ernie, Ed, and others get their start. It entails little risk of injury and may be seen as an exciting challenge, especially among groups of children who spur each other on.

Sophisticated young thieves may use stolen credit cards or checkbooks, and some keep pace with technology by turning to computer and electronic crime. Images of young computer hackers sneaking past electronic sentries have become commonplace, and some of these troublemakers have long histories of misbehavior. I recall an IBM advertisement that played on this idea to sell information security, voicing a fear ascribed to today's executives: "Will a 14-year-old sociopath bring my company to its knees?" Children with conduct disorder, like adult antisocials, can be extremely adaptable, jumping at any opportunity to make mischief or to get what they want.

BREAKING THE RULES

Serious violations of rules, the fourth area of major problem behaviors, often are noted in schools, if not at home. The structure and demands of learning provide ample opportunity for troubled children to rebel, and teachers may be the first to identify "problem" kids with severe behavior disorders. Rule violations and poor school performance—worse than predicted by measures of intelligence—lead to high rates of failure, truancy, suspension, and permanent expulsion. These problems are of enormous importance because they stunt educational achievement, contribute to future job difficulties, and set the stage for low income and social status in adulthood.

Evidence of trouble in today's schools—metal detectors installed at the doors, reports of "sexting," and drug activity—all contribute to an impression that students are becoming increasingly brazen, but the vast majority of kids do not display the behaviors associated with conduct disorder beyond a few minor transgressions. Perhaps the most chilling reminder that school has become an increasingly dangerous place is the growing number of school shootings. The shootings at Columbine High School, located outside Denver, in 1999, were particularly shocking. Two senior students—Dylan Klebold and Eric Harris—killed 13 people, injured an additional 24, and then killed themselves. The two had a history of juvenile delinquency, including making death threats and felony theft. Few would have ever guessed the extent of their anger toward society that led to the senseless shootings.[11]

The home, too, is the setting for rule violations like missed curfews, running away, or simply ignoring parental instructions. Children with conduct disorder can test the patience, will, and courage of even the most competent parents, especially as they grow older and become more difficult to control. In 1996, a Michigan couple was fined under a local ordinance requiring that parents "exercise reasonable control over their minor children," a law resembling those enacted in other communities and states.[12] The couple's 16-year-old son had burglarized several churches, attacked his father with a golf club, and refused counseling. He was later sentenced to a year in juvenile detention on burglary, weapons, and drug charges after his troubled parents—who feared for the safety of the boy's two younger sisters—cooperated with police. Local authorities had urged the couple to assert control over their son, which is easier said than done with a violent boy four inches taller than his father. I have worked with parents in similar situations and respect the challenges they face, as children with conduct disorder can be frustratingly uncontrollable and even fearsome.

But, in many cases, parents themselves contribute to their children's bad behavior through abuse or neglect. Take Yummy, for example. His mother, one of 10 children from four different fathers, gave birth to eight children herself, the first when she was 15. She left Yummy's father because of his bad temper and was charged with neglect after one of her children went blind from an untreated eye condition. Yummy was treated for suspicious injuries before age two and reportedly was found covered with burns and welts a year later, when the children were removed from the home after neighbors complained that they were left unattended. (The mother denied ever beating her children.) Yummy and the others were placed with their grandmother, whom psychiatrists described as domineering and emotionally unstable. While this chaotic home life and other environmental factors do not excuse or completely explain Yummy's short life of crime, research repeatedly shows that parental neglect and abuse have profound, lifelong effects. Parents—some undeniably antisocial—who shirk their responsibilities or abuse their children, contribute to an ongoing, multigenerational cycle of violence and other problems. In later chapters, I will discuss how a lax or abusive home environment can be a factor in the transmission of ASP from parent to child.

THE CHILD IS FATHER OF THE MAN

A history of conduct disorder observed during childhood or noted after the fact is one of four necessary criteria for a diagnosis of adult ASP as defined by the *DSM-IV-TR*. Not all children with conduct disorder grow up to become antisocial, but those who do—about 40% of boys and 25% of girls with conduct disorder—continue their pattern of misbehavior on an adult scale.[13] The most important criterion for ASP is a pervasive disregard for the rights of others, characterized by some of the same signs that define conduct disorder: failure to conform with social norms and standards of lawful behavior, deceit, impulsiveness or failure to plan ahead, irritability and aggressiveness, reckless disregard for the safety of oneself and others, consistent irresponsibility, and lack of remorse. An ASP diagnosis also requires that the individual in question be at least 18 years old and that antisocial behavior not occur exclusively during the course of schizophrenia or a manic episode.

The latter two criteria caution psychiatrists not to be too quick in diagnosing ASP. By requiring that the diagnosis be applied only to those older than 18, *DSM-IV-TR* discourages labeling young people with a serious diagnosis that may remain a troublesome aspect of their medical records even if later proven wrong or if their problems subside. The final criterion demands that other serious mental disorders with symptoms that can mimic those of ASP be ruled out as causes for bad behavior. Schizophrenia, for example, can cause personality changes, hallucinations and delusions, and bizarre behavior. Mania, an extreme state of elation and excitation that occurs in persons with bipolar (or manic-depressive) illness, can cause irritability, aggression, excessive sexual impulses, and hyperactivity, bringing an array of irrational and hurtful behaviors that stem from a treatable mood disorder rather than a longstanding personality disturbance.

Perhaps the most significant aspect of ASP is the way antisocials repeatedly ignore and violate the rights of others, engaging in destructive, criminal, and sometimes brutal acts. *DSM-IV-TR* defines this pattern with seven categories of symptoms. For a diagnosis of ASP to apply, a patient must exhibit problems in at least three of these categories, although, in my experience, most antisocials meet all seven criteria. To make the diagnosis, mental health professionals seek out clues from interviews with patients and families, medical and legal documents, and other sources. With ASP, the signs may emerge quite readily.

THE DSM-IV-TR CRITERIA FOR ANTISOCIAL PERSONALITY DISORDER ARE:

A. There is a pervasive pattern of disregard for and violation of the rights of others occurring since age 15 years indicated by three or more of the following:

1. Failure to conform to social norms with respect to lawful behaviors as indicated by repeatedly performing acts that are grounds for arrest

2. Deceitfulness, as indicated by repeated lying, use of aliases, or conning of others for personal profit or pleasure

3. Impulsivity or failure to plan ahead

4. Irritability and aggressiveness, as indicated by repeated physical fights or assaults

5. Reckless disregard for safety of others or self

6. Consistent irresponsibility, as indicated by repeated failure to sustain consistent work behavior or honor financial obligations

7. Lack of remorse, as indicated by being indifferent to or rationalizing having hurt, mistreated, or stolen from another

B. The individual is at least 18 years.

C. There is evidence of Conduct Disorder with onset before age 15 years.

D. The occurrence of antisocial behavior is not exclusively during the course of Schizophrenia or a Manic Episode.

(Reprinted with permission from the *Diagnostic and Statistical Manual of Mental Disorders*, 4th ed. Text Revision. Copyright 2000, American Psychiatric Association.)

In my mind, the variety of bad behaviors that characterize ASP make the disorder easy to identify, a process I take up in the next chapter. However, individual symptoms sometimes take precedence over others, distracting psychiatrists and other mental health professionals from the diagnosis, or ASP is masked by a coexisting condition, like alcoholism. Antisocial personality disorder is a blend of acts and attitudes, and how a patient views his behavior is as important as the behavior itself. For many antisocials, lack of conscience enables them to act on impulses without a second thought and then to repeat the same destructive behaviors with no regard for their consequences. Although antisocials can understand the concepts of right and wrong on an intellectual level, they have no emotional connection to commonly held standards of behavior. This conscience deficit is the root of ASP's range of symptoms.

FAILURE TO CONFORM

Legal records often substantiate an ASP diagnosis, so the first criterion, a failure to conform to social norms and laws, is especially important. As predictably as night follows day, most antisocials have trouble with the law. From theft, forgery, and embezzlement, to drug dealing and robbery, to sexual attacks and other acts of violence, antisocial adults may take their childhood offenses to terrible extremes. Most often, however, their criminal records are notable not for their savagery, but for their sheer length and variety. Because so many antisocials are addicted to drugs or alcohol, their crimes often revolve around substance abuse, whether committed in a haze of intoxication or out of a need to acquire the drug of choice. Such behaviors are often behind the individual's arrests, convictions, and incarceration. According to Lee Robins in *Deviant Children Grown Up*, nearly three-quarters of antisocials spend one or more years behind bars.[14]

Almost 40% are incarcerated for five years or more. In my own research, 75% of antisocial men were arrested multiple times, and 48% had been convicted of a felony.

The types of criminal histories that support an ASP diagnosis may vary, but psychiatrists who are accustomed to dealing with the disorder are quick to spot its telltale signs. When I hear about a man like Jerry Lee Proctor, convicted of the 1994 kidnapping, rape, and murder of a Des Moines woman, I wonder what might have happened had someone paid close attention to his criminal record, one that resembles those of many antisocials.[15] In 1985, he was charged with assault causing bodily injury. The following year, he was accused of assaulting his mother, damaging her car and home, interfering with police, and possessing marijuana. In 1991, he was given a one-year suspended sentence for domestic assault causing injury, and then was charged with threatening to kill the girlfriend he had attacked. His 1992 charges included third-degree criminal mischief, assault with intent to commit sexual abuse, and interference with official acts. In 1995, he was fined for simple misdemeanor assault. Although this history did not predict that he would become a killer, it should have raised some concern, something that advocates for battered women and rape victims pointed out after Proctor's arrest on murder charges.

It does not take a history of violence to suggest ASP. The story of Kevin Mitnick, a computer hacker apprehended in 1995, raised my suspicions when I read it in the national press.[16] He started breaking into computer networks as a teenager, first snooping through his high school's administrative system. Soon, he turned his attention to telephone systems and was caught stealing technical manuals from Pacific Bell's computers, a crime that earned him probation. He spent six months in jail after breaking into a university system, and later served a one-year prison sentence for stealing proprietary computer codes. After undergoing treatment for "computer addiction," he was ordered to steer clear of computers and modems, but the temptation was apparently too great to resist. Implicated in additional crimes, he spent three years on the run before being captured with $1 million in stolen data and charged with computer fraud and illegal use of a telephone access device. Mitnick was diagnosed with obsessive-compulsive disorder and depression by the psychotherapist who attempted to treat his supposed addiction, but his pattern of criminality is not unlike that associated with ASP.

DECEIT

Deceit is another significant way in which antisocials display their disregard for others. Many are able to craft an elaborate system of lies in pursuit of their aims or in an effort to escape responsibility. The con men we hear about—for instance, those who prey on elderly homeowners with unnecessary "repair" schemes or others who separate the sick from their savings with phony remedies—display a seemingly innate ability to pervert the truth.

Terms like *compulsive* or *pathological liar* may prove apt descriptions for many people with ASP, whose lies vary according to the situation. An antisocial man bucking for a better job may falsify his work record; another seeking to explain a five-day absence to his wife may invent a whopper about kidnapping. Or an antisocial may concoct a story for his own amusement, attempting to impress friends, relatives, or drinking companions. These creative fictions may trace great achievements, brushes with famous people, or heroic deeds. A young man expelled from Yale was charged with accepting more than $60,000 in loans and scholarships under false pretenses after authorities discovered that he had forged his academic record and transfer application to the prestigious university.[17] He inflated his grade point average, supplied recommendations from nonexistent teachers, falsified his high school transcript, and even boasted of being related to a well-known actor. The scheme was worthy of the craftiest antisocial. Although psychotic patients may actually believe the delusional stories they tell, antisocials know full well that their stories are lies.

Many antisocials, including the infamous serial killer Ted Bundy, find that escaping responsibility or pulling off crimes is easier when they adopt a string of aliases. Some antisocials seem to change their names nearly as often as they change their clothing, frustrating those with reason to follow their trails. Like Ernie, in the last chapter, these men take up aliases to gain freedom from past obligations and evade law enforcement, creditors, or former spouses. Others assume false names to facilitate con games. One recent story mirrors the play and film *Six Degrees of Separation* (itself inspired by an actual event), in which a wealthy family is duped by a man who claims to be the son of actor Sidney Poitier. In a recent real-life version, a convicted criminal with a history of forgery and theft posed as a prominent academic to rook professors at colleges across the country out of more than $200,000.[18] He would telephone, drop a famous name, and ask his "colleagues" to loan various sums to a nonexistent nephew. Later, he would arrive to pick up the cash, this time posing as the down-on-his-luck relative. Although his scheme seems farfetched, it was surprisingly successful.

IMPULSIVENESS

Antisocials tend to be impulsive, unable to see beyond their immediate circumstances or learn from past rash actions. Decisions are made quickly, often without reflection or consideration of possible outcomes. Like Cleckley's psychopaths, antisocials rarely follow a life plan and instead live for the moment. The word *wanderlust* is used to describe persons who move from place to place without any particular goal or destination, but it might also help them dodge past crimes and identities. Like Ed, whose story is told in this chapter, antisocials frequently cite pursuit of "a fresh start" as justification for taking to the road. In his book *Shot in the Heart*, Mikal Gilmore portrays the aimless wanderings of his con-man father, Frank, and hapless mother, Bessie, who usually left when the law got too close: "They would move into a place, spend a couple of weeks and then move on. Rarely did they stay anyplace for as long as a month or two and when the time came to leave, it was almost always in a hurry.... As it turned out, there were often good reasons for moving on quickly. Frank's main career, Bessie began to see, was scamming ... selling advertising for a forthcoming magazine ... [that] would never materialize."[19]

Like the runaway child, the antisocial adult may leave for days at a time, telling no one where he has been or what he has done. Was it an alcoholic bender? A sexual dalliance? A crime spree? Or was it sheer escapism, a reminder of the freedom attained by shirking all obligations? Some antisocials seem to feed on the excitement of escape, the way the road tests their wits, and may perhaps make it a way of life. Whether we call them hoboes, vagrants, or nomads, these men—like Paul Mendez, whose story appeared in Chapter 1—seem to prefer their peripatetic lives to the workaday drudgery of maintaining a job, home, and responsibility to family. Wounded while serving with the U.S. Army in Vietnam, Mendez estimated having visited 40 states during 15 years of riding freight trains. "I want to see what I fought for," he told a reporter after eight double whiskeys with beer chasers. "I fought for you, mister. I fought for this whole country ... I fought for the United States of America."[20] Although many of us think of homeless men as victims of poverty, addiction, or psychoses—and many are—some are antisocial, driven to the streets by desire rather than despair. In fact, studies in St. Louis and Los Angeles show that about 25% of the homeless are antisocial.[21] The antisocial may prefer to take life as it comes, without the plans that most of us form. Of course, his failure to plan ahead or adhere to the demands of education and employment may limit his economic and social resources, perhaps keeping success elusive even for those who eventually settle down. Nevertheless, we do antisocials a disservice when we consider them little more than prisoners of their disorder. These men are often well aware of their choices. Unfortunately, many of them consistently pick the wrong ones.

AGGRESSION

The most disturbing symptom of ASP is aggression, expressed in shades from quiet intimidation to explosive violence. The aggressive antisocial is dangerous. His actions may be sudden and unpredictable, but more likely they are deliberate, purposeful, and designed for maximum impact. In mild cases, the antisocial is simply irritable, occasionally lashing out at family, co-workers, or strangers. But in other cases, even the most minor disputes rapidly escalate to brutality. Domestic violence is common in the families of these men, creating a climate of terror for spouses and children, who live in fear of the next outburst, knowing that the attacks often stem from no apparent cause. Violent antisocials often end up in jail, which may be the best place for them. As family members and other victims of antisocial violence can attest, these men should be avoided at all costs.

This is not to say that aggression is always a hindrance for antisocials, breeding violence that lands them behind bars. Some are able to escape the law, whereas others channel their violent tendencies in directions that earn approval or success. Some become successful boxers, wrestlers, or soldiers, although most lack the discipline or tolerance for the regulations that such occupations require. I would not profess to diagnose Mike Tyson with ASP or any other condition, but his history reveals the aggressive tendencies associated with antisocial personality.[22] Growing up on the streets of Brooklyn, Tyson was apprehended several times before age 12 for mugging and robbery. He developed the combative talents that would later bring him fame and wealth as a boxer, but Tyson had an unpredictable violent streak. A former wife complained that he was violent and hot tempered and, in 1992, he was convicted of raping an 18-year-old beauty pageant contestant (a charge he denied). Tyson spent three years behind bars, but returned to boxing after his 1995 release. Two years later, he was suspended from the sport after biting off part of Evander Holyfield's ear during a match. Violence continued to dog him. In 1999, he attempted to break both arms of boxer François Botha, and he returned to prison later that year for having assaulted two motorists following a traffic accident the prior year. He retired from boxing in 2005, but continues to have highly publicized problems that include marital infidelity, illegal drug use, and traffic violations. He recently told talk show host Ellen DeGeneres that he has improved his life by becoming sober and adopting a vegan diet.

RECKLESSNESS

Antisocials' disregard for others and for themselves is expressed in subtler ways as well. Many show a symptomatic recklessness, driving too fast or while drunk, practicing unsafe sex, or taking countless other risks. As I have already noted, accidents and traumatic injuries from fights may limit the lifespan of many antisocials.[23] In fact, people with ASP are also more likely to be murdered, prompting a theory that the apparent burnout in older antisocials may be caused by a tendency for the worst ones to be killed off early in life.[24] If they survive to old age, many antisocials display health problems, the result of ignoring illness, delaying medical care, or simply failing to follow through on treatment recommendations. It is no wonder that antisocials have higher than normal death rates from diseases that require careful management, such as diabetes and human immunodeficiency virus (HIV) infection. HIV/AIDS and other sexually transmitted diseases are common among antisocials, and the reckless approach that many of them take to sex puts unsuspecting partners at risk.[25]

IRRESPONSIBILITY

Irresponsibility enters every aspect of an antisocial's life, from work and finances to family and social relations. The employment histories of antisocials often reveal telltale inconsistencies: periods of unemployment, a tendency to take on part-time work that seldom lasts, frequent job changes. An antisocial may begin a job with great energy but soon lose interest. Then the problems begin. First, he is late, then misses work without good reason. He may lie about his hours, fail to complete assigned tasks, slack off or even sleep on the job, and take time off when expected to work. Arguments or fights with co-workers or supervisors may erupt and, when confronted about his poor performance, the antisocial summons ready excuses. If he is not fired, his lack of interest or frustration with the demands of employment may drive him to quit abruptly, often without any alternative source of support. Irresponsibility combined with work problems create tenuous financial situations for many antisocials, who prefer to spend whatever money remains on yet one more drink, another lotto ticket, or that last lap dance. Credit tends to be poor, substantial debts accumulate, and many end up on public assistance or charity.

Some antisocials do better in jobs with little direct supervision or when self-employed, where the demands of others are relatively few and less likely to prompt resistance in those unaccustomed to following any sort of regulation. They may remain at work longer as truck drivers, or as traveling sales and service representatives, jobs that permit a degree of independence and keep the antisocial on the road. Some pursue illegal occupations, such as drug dealing, pimping, or prostitution. In the 1950s, Lee Robins found that the jobs held longest by antisocials tended to involve drinking or serving as fronts for illegal activity.[26] She noted that antisocials often work as bartenders, waiters, entertainers, hotel bellhops, or carnival workers. Of course, antisocials are found across the social and economic spectrum, and some, aided by above-average intelligence, wealth, or connections, manage to escape the downward spiral in employment. Antisocial personality disorder is found everywhere and in every profession, including medicine, law, politics, and the clergy. Of the subjects followed in my research study, one became a lawyer (although he was eventually disbarred), three joined the clergy, and several became psychotherapists.

Relationships and family life are another area in which irresponsibility becomes a dominant feature. Many antisocials marry young, divorce freely, and remarry several times during their lives. As with a new job, each budding relationship may start with high hopes for both the antisocial and his partner. The liaisons that prompt many marriages with antisocials are often too short to expose anything beyond the antisocial's façade of normalcy, but the deeper truth soon emerges. After a few months, fear and intimidation are sometimes the strongest bonds at work in the relationship. Verbal, physical, and sexual abuse erupt, and infidelity introduces additional health risks. The relationship problems encountered by many antisocials may be due in part to their tendency to become involved with equally unstable partners. One study of female felons found that three-quarters had married antisocial men,[27] providing evidence that, at least in the case of antisocials, like tends to seek out like.

Antisocials often make incompetent parents. When children are involved, the antisocial's irresponsibility affects the entire family, perpetuating a wide range of problems. People with ASP are much more likely to abuse or neglect their children than are others. In fact, in one study, antisocials were seven times more likely to abuse their children than were non-antisocials, and more than 12 times more likely to neglect them.[28] Antisocials may be unwilling or unable to provide necessary economic support for their offspring, condemning the children to the hardship of poverty. The antisocial man who divorces or leaves the home cannot be counted on for much of anything, and some of the men we now call "deadbeat dads" are no doubt antisocial. Efforts by states to collect unpaid child and spousal support may contribute yet another offense to the lengthy legal records of many people with ASP. A *New York Times* article about women on welfare profiled one mother whose situation is all too familiar.[29] At age 14, she was seduced by a married man in his early 30s, and the two of them saw each other for almost two years before she became pregnant. She eventually had four children with the man, whom she described as behaving the way many antisocials do. He floated in and out of her life at his convenience, sometimes beating her, never holding a steady job, ignoring his responsibilities to their children. Despite all this, she claimed to still love him.

Consistent irresponsibility also contributes to a lack of social relationships among antisocials.[30] Relationships that develop tend to be shallow, perhaps based on shared affinities for drink or drugs rather than anything more meaningful. Communication is not a priority for many antisocials and, in most social activities, the less of it, the better. Antisocials rarely join community organizations, volunteer agencies, or church groups, although some turn up at Alcoholics Anonymous or other recovery groups, especially when motivated by a court order. Some antisocials who do become involved in their communities may have ulterior motives—for example, the antisocial pedophile who works as a volunteer for organizations that permit contact with young children.

LACK OF REMORSE

Related to irresponsibility is the antisocial's seeming inability to feel regret or remorse for his actions. This lack of conscience traps antisocials in emotional isolation, underlies their disregard for all standards of behavior, and dooms them to live without the social support that most of us take for granted. But many antisocials wouldn't have it any other way. They see themselves as the true victims, not those they betray, rob, rape, or murder. They hold a perpetual grudge against the social order and inspire outrage when they reveal the contorted logic that, in their eyes, absolves them of all responsibility. We see this symptom of ASP in the news accounts of criminal defendants who express no shame for their crimes and make no apologies. Whether motivated by a sincere belief in their self-proclaimed victimhood or by a deliberate desire to offend, these men thumb their noses at those they hurt. Research confirms that lack of remorse is particularly common with more severe and violent forms of ASP, perhaps allowing men like killer John Wayne Gacy, who is profiled in Chapter 9, to maintain an attitude of defiance that helps seal their fate.[31] Up to the day of his execution, Gacy denied involvement in the murders of 33 men whose bodies were found beneath his house and lawn. He even considered writing a book titled *The 34th Victim*.[32] I read about another convicted criminal, a repeat sex offender, who similarly rejected all responsibility for his crimes. Rather than denying the charges, he placed blame squarely on his victims: "I get around teenagers, and they take advantage of me, and the next thing I know, I'm in trouble."[33]

Another example is Jack Abbott, a convicted murderer who forged a quixotic relationship with author Norman Mailer.[34] Abbott's letters to the writer depicted prison life in an intense and direct style, prompting Mailer to assist in publishing a collection of the writings called *In the Belly of the Beast*, which Abbott dedicated to serial killer Carl Panzram. In the foreword, Mailer describes Abbott's long history behind bars, his life as a self-described "state-raised convict." Abbott's rambling account omits any mention of the crimes that sent him to prison, but he takes every opportunity to portray himself as a victim, caught in a web of unjust laws. "After all this that society has done, I am naturally resentful," he writes. "I don't want revenge; to punish. I just would like an apology of some sort. A little consideration. Just a small recognition by society of the injustice that has been done to me, not to mention others like me." Abbott was eventually released from prison, due in part to the efforts of Mailer and other supporters. Just six weeks later, he fatally stabbed a waiter, after a restaurant altercation, and was convicted of manslaughter. He returned to prison, where he committed suicide with a makeshift noose fashioned from bed sheets and shoelaces.

THE ANTISOCIAL WOMAN: AN EQUAL OPPORTUNITY DISORDER

Antisocial personality is a man's disorder, but it would be incorrect to conclude that women don't develop ASP, because many do. Although the book's title focuses attention on the fact that some bad boys become bad men, bad girls sometimes become bad women, but they do so at much lower rates than men. Why does this gender difference come as a surprise to some? In fact, many psychiatric disorders are more common in one gender. Schizophrenia, alcoholism, drug addictions, and ADHD are more frequent in men, whereas depression, anxiety disorders, somatization, and borderline personality disorder are more common in women. These gender gaps raise important questions about the reasons behind them. Most theories involve diagnostic practices that may favor one gender, genetics, hormones, social environment, or some combination of these various possibilities, but no one really knows.

Lee Robins described women antisocials in *Deviant Children Grown Up*. In childhood, troubled girls later diagnosed as antisocial resembled boys with similar diagnoses, except that they were more likely to have had sexual misbehavior and to have a later onset of behavioral problems. As women, they married at a younger age than their non-antisocial peers and chose husbands "who drank, were arrested, were unfaithful, deserted, or failed to support them. When choosing a second husband, at a more mature age, they showed little evidence from having profited from their mistakes."[35] Those with children had more of them than did non-antisocial women, and their children tended to be difficult, perhaps sadly destined to follow their parents' path in life. Like her male counterpart, the woman antisocial has trouble with low earnings and financial dependency, and she engages in aggressive behavior. These women are disconnected from the community and have high rates of depression, anxiety disorders, and addiction.[36]

Other data on gender differences suggest that antisocial boys are more likely than antisocial girls to engage in fighting, use weapons, engage in cruelty to animals, or set fires. Girls are more often involved in "victimless" antisocial behaviors, such as running away. As adults, women with ASP are more likely to have problems that center on the home and family, such as irresponsibility as a parent, neglectful or abusive treatment of their children, and being physically violent toward husbands and partners.[37] If one looks to crime statistics as an indicator of differences, women clearly are less likely to be convicted and incarcerated for violent crimes than are men.[38]

Troubled women are fodder for the tabloids, but truly antisocial women are less common and therefore noteworthy when they appear in the news. One such case that transfixed the nation was that of Sante Kimes. And, although Kimes' behavior is extreme, and she is not representative, her symptoms are undeniably antisocial. For many years, she and her son Kenneth were a tag team of lies, cons, arson, forgery, theft, and, eventually, murder. In the book *Son of a Grifter*, estranged son Kent Walker describes how Kimes' forte was fleecing people of money through elaborate schemes that often involved insurance fraud, in which she committed arson to collect for property damage.[39] But she also committed offenses that had no obvious financial gain, such as enslaving maids—who were often illegal immigrants—when she could afford to pay them, or burning down houses she could have sold. She and son Kenneth were arrested in 1998 for the death of their landlady, New York socialite Irene Silverman. Sante planned to assume her identity and take ownership of her $7.7 million Manhattan mansion. The mother and son couple were convicted, even though Silverman's body was never found. Kenneth had confessed to strangling Silverman after Sante had "tased" the woman; the two later disposed of the body in a Hoboken, New Jersey dumpster. During the sentencing portion of the trial, Sante made a lengthy statement to the court blaming the authorities for framing her, and compared the trial to the Salem Witch Trials. The presiding judge declared her a "sociopath" and "remorseless predator." She was later convicted in a 2004 trial in Los Angeles for the murder of a man who had threatened to expose Kimes in a forgery scheme in Las Vegas in the 1990s. Both Sante and Kenneth are serving life in prison, she in New York, he in California.

Critics have suggested that at least some of the gender gap in ASP may be the result of biased criteria. Because women are less apt to commit violent crimes and less likely to be arrested than men, they are also less likely to meet the *DSM-IV-TR* criteria because these criteria favor typically male patterns of problem behaviors.[40] If so, then the gender differences are an artifact of gender bias. I personally believe the difference is true, because virtually all research studies have shown this gender split, in spite of their differing methods, samples, and diagnostic criteria.

Genetics could play a role as well. Wendy Slutske, a behavioral geneticist at the University of Missouri, points out that, on balance, antisocial women have *more* genetic risk factors (as well as non-genetic factors that run in families, such as abuse and neglect) than do antisocial men, meaning that women require more family risk factors—genetic and nongenetic—before they become antisocial.[41] She says: "In other words, it may be more difficult to produce an antisocial woman than an antisocial man."

Another possibility, as some have maintained, is that because some antisocial women express their personality disorder through promiscuous sex or emotionally manipulative relationships, the psychiatrist instead makes the diagnosis *borderline personality disorder*. People with borderline personality disorder have unstable moods, impulsive behaviors, and sometimes commit self-damaging acts (like cutting one's wrists). Although there is some overlap, borderline personality disorder and ASP are fundamentally different: ASP is characterized by acting-out behaviors, whereas people with borderline personality disorder tend to turn their emotions inward.

With continued shifts in gender norms, we might expect to see more women diagnosed with ASP in the future. We see this already in the prison system where I consult and conduct research. The percentage of men and women diagnosed as antisocial is nearly the same, meaning that, at least in this setting, irresponsible, deceitful, or aggressive behavior should suggest ASP regardless of gender.[42]

THE DIAGNOSIS, THEN AND NOW

The symptoms of ASP are expressed in a range of actions and attitudes that may not themselves be recognized as warning signs.

Addiction or other health conditions can disguise ASP as the source of trouble, diverting attention from the common cause behind an antisocial's spectrum of misbehavior. Aggression and irresponsibility, or any other qualities that define the disorder, may be seen as isolated symptoms, obscuring the relationship between antisocial traits. Again, it is a long-term pattern of misbehavior that characterizes ASP. Unfortunately, this telltale pattern is often glimpsed only in fragments, giving infrequent observers a misimpression. The case studies in this book provide examples of how the disorder manifests and illustrate the many similarities between cases. But each antisocial is unique. Some are capable of savage violence, whereas others appear relatively harmless, at least to those who don't fall victim to their swindles, cons, or broken promises. Ed is one man whose life, although punctuated with occasional violence, followed a path of petty crime, disappearances, and manipulation.

Ed spent nine days in the hospital following his 1950 admission, eventually demanding to be discharged against his doctor's advice. The psychiatrist had found him physically normal, "a lightly built man appearing younger than his stated age." He wrote that Ed was "well oriented in all spheres and shows no defects in remote or recent memory," and that he showed no abnormalities of speech or language. At one point, Ed confessed to his problems and pondered an explanation, describing himself as "a maladjusted case" and wondering whether he was unduly influenced by a corrupt subconscious. The doctor paid little attention to his patient's theory, scribbling a note about Ed's ability to describe unpleasant material from his past without batting an eye. The true diagnosis, in the doctor's eyes, was "psychopathic personality," then the current term.

Forty years later, my colleagues and I set out to find Ed. Cathy Butler began with his hometown telephone directory, then moved on to the Iowa State Division of Motor Vehicles, which provided an address in Des Moines. A letter sent there was returned unopened, without a forwarding address. Credit bureau traces produced two different Arizona addresses, but letters sent to them also came back unclaimed. The Social Security Administration had an address on file and willingly forwarded our letter, but we received no response. Despite the frustrating series of failures, we at least learned that Ed was alive. From his 1950 hospital chart, we knew he had a younger brother, so Cathy returned to the hometown phone directory, calling every Honneker in the book. Eventually, she landed an important lead, an elderly woman who referred her to a friend in the local nursing home. The friend reportedly had relatives named Honneker, and Cathy hoped she wasn't headed for yet another dead end. Her call to the home was received by a woman who, although suspicious of Cathy's motives, admitted to being Ed's maternal aunt. By amazing coincidence, Ed's brother Peter was visiting her that day.

Peter hadn't spoken to Ed in years and had no idea where he could be found. Although he agreed to talk with Cathy about his brother, he postponed the conversation to spare his elderly aunt the grief of learning all her elder nephew's failings. In passing, he mentioned that Ed had experienced a difficult series of financial troubles and run-ins with the law, and perhaps still lived in Arizona, although he couldn't be sure. It was an encouraging start for Cathy, who arranged to contact Peter weeks later. We were never able to locate Ed, but his brother provided the details needed to construct a history of Ed's life. Sometime after his hospital discharge in 1950, Ed had managed to return to the West, only to vanish from his family and from us. He would have been 66 years old at the time of my study.

Ed was a family disgrace, but Peter, like his father, was a respected judge. He had followed his father in another way as well, by helping to rescue Ed in times of trouble, at least at first. After years of fielding calls from angry creditors, Peter had given up on his brother and let their relationship wither. His only news of Ed's doings came from frequent collection calls, mostly from credit card companies that had made the mistake of approving Ed's applications. Peter couldn't help them. He had realized years before that Ed was an accomplished con artist who would take advantage of anyone who let him. Although his father had never given up hope, Peter could no longer be so forgiving.

According to Peter, Ed had headed to Arizona after his arrest in 1950, settling in Tucson, continuing his education at the state university, and marrying for the second time. After graduating, he returned to Iowa with his new wife and entered law school, apparently intent on following in his father's footsteps. The judge and his wife tempered their pride with caution but were unable to resist the hope that Ed had reformed and was finally going to make it. Ed received his degree—in fact, doing quite well—and his wife gave birth to their first child. But trouble returned when the state bar association rejected Ed's application for admission, citing his criminal past. Ed spiraled into his old pattern of drinking and domestic strife, threatening his wife while consumed by alcoholic rage. She left him and filed for divorce. Peter recalled her anguished lament that she could no longer stand Ed's "running around with other women, lack of responsibility, spending money carelessly, having an attention span of about three months, and living in his own little dream world."

Despite the divorce and his tussles with drink, Ed kept petitioning the bar for admission until his persistence paid off. He established a solo practice in Des Moines, once again making a vigorous start that proved to be short-lived. Returning to his old ways, he forged checks in a client's name and was disbarred for three years, then fled the state and assumed an alias to escape criminal prosecution. After two years on the lam, he was apprehended and extradited back to Iowa, but his family connections spared him a state prison sentence. By the time Ed was returned to Iowa, however, he was a chronic alcoholic.

At this point, Peter's details became vague as he recounted Ed's habit of drifting in and out of sight. He had fathered two children in his first two marriages, but neither ever knew him. Once the divorces were settled, his earliest wives never spoke to Ed again, but Peter could not attest to the women his brother had known in later years. He estimated that Ed had married four or five times, and he told Cathy that Ed's latest wife was 23 years his junior. Handsome and well dressed regardless of his circumstances, his brother was able to manipulate many women—and some men—with his charm. Cathy noted Peter's disgust as he described Ed's pathological lying: "Almost nothing Ed says can be believed. He's a definite con artist."

Peter had little doubt that Ed was still finding his way into legal trouble, although he knew it had been more than a decade since his last arrest in Iowa. Ed's records confirmed his brother's account, listing 14 arrests between 1942 and 1967, mostly for forgery but with one aggravated assault. When Ed and his wife visited Iowa, Peter ran a police trace on the car they were driving and later found it had been stolen from the Phoenix airport. Ed left before Peter could confront him but not before running up a huge long distance bill on Peter's phone. Peter remarked with some relief that Ed's visits home were infrequent and seldom included important family events. In fact, he had missed his mother's funeral.

Cathy asked Peter whether his brother had ever held any goals. Peter thought for a moment, then responded that Ed's sole ambition had been respect and notoriety. He wanted to be recognized, honored, even emulated. As it turned out, his only fame had come in small-town police departments and whispered gossip among neighbors and family friends. Although Peter thought Ed was little more than a drifter and a self-described "amateur historian," he recalled that his brother had recently mentioned something about selling aluminum siding under an assumed name—"easier for customers to spell," Ed had claimed. With a mixture of disgust and regret, Peter added, "It's a damn shame that a person as intelligent and funny as Ed couldn't make a life for himself."

Ed's story bears many earmarks of ASP: his repeated arrests on criminal charges, constant lies to his family, his frequent flights in the face of trouble, a spotty work history, the abandonment of his children and past wives. It also shows how family and friends, no matter how well meaning, can unwittingly enable antisocial behavior in those with ASP. People like Ed learn during childhood how to manipulate others in the way most of us learn to tie our shoes or ride a bicycle. Their early habits become second nature, valuable tools for living beyond society's grasp. It is possible that early intervention and the full brunt of the law might have helped Ed mend his ways, but as I will show, the course of ASP often seems to have been determined very early. Ed's case is not one of "falling off the wagon," as he told his psychiatrist in 1950. He never got on.

Chapter 4

Naming the Problem

The Diagnosis of
Antisocial Personality Disorder

PAUL'S CASE

Driving through a suburban neighborhood, Paul Olsen, age 54, spotted a young girl on her way home from school. He slowed the car and pulled up to the curb, motioning to her and mentioning something vague about directions. As she approached, Paul opened his pants, exposed his penis, and began to masturbate. The horrified girl turned and ran to the nearest house, and Paul sped away from the scene. But he was not quick enough to evade the sharp eyes of a passing driver and, hours later, the police caught up with him at a bar near his home. He was arrested for exhibitionism, and a judge ordered him to receive a psychiatric evaluation at the hospital where I practice.

Paul showed signs of alcohol withdrawal when I met him on the psychiatric ward. He was disheveled, sweat beaded on his brow, and his feet beat out a jittery rhythm on the tile floor. He readily confessed to having an unusual sexual appetite, a taste for girls "of a certain size," between the ages of 11 and 14. He admitted six to eight occasions when he had approached such girls and exposed himself, claiming that the episodes provided "tension relief" for a drive fueled by alcohol and a sizable collection of pornography. I suspected that his true number of encounters was substantially higher. Unlike most pedophiles, who desire physical contact with prepubescent children, Paul said exhibitionism was enough for him. He delighted in the shock his behavior produced, and each experience provided enough fantasy material to sustain him for a while. Eventually, however, he would return to the prowl, often while drunk. His most recent venture had brought his first arrest for a sexual offense.

Paul did not seem particularly anxious or upset over the behavior itself, although clearly he was concerned about getting back to the streets and to his favorite bottle. I noted his complete lack of remorse and the defiant tone he assumed. Paul seemed driven as much by a desire to offend as by the pursuit of sexual thrills. He enjoyed not only the fear he saw in the faces of his young victims, but also the way his behavior violated social taboos and legal strictures. Almost immediately, I sensed something more to Paul's case than a paraphilia—the psychiatric term for sexual deviance. He was clearly troubled, whether he knew it or not, and I suspected that a thorough psychiatric evaluation would reveal a man who lived his life against the grain of society.

THE CHALLENGE OF DIAGNOSIS

Very few people seek psychiatric attention or counseling specifically for antisocial personality disorder (ASP), and antisocials generally scoff at the idea that they might have a significant illness. Yet in the Epidemiologic Catchment Area (ECA) study, nearly 20% of antisocials had sought mental health care in the past year, whereas a recent study in the United Kingdom showed that nearly 25% had done so.[1] Antisocials are prompted to seek care by particularly troublesome symptoms, such as domestic violence, excessive alcohol or drug use, or suicidal behavior, often leaving the underlying problem of ASP undiscovered. Other antisocials only submit to evaluation at the demand of family members or the courts and then resist cooperation. Those who begin treatment—whether voluntarily or not—and thus learn something about ASP often reject the diagnosis, denying its symptoms and the possibility that it might be responsible for their troubles. Someone else always has the problem, never them.

Cleckley described this "specific loss of insight," the inability to assess one's own feelings and behavior rationally: "In a special sense, the psychopath lacks insight to a degree seldom, if ever found in any but the most seriously disturbed psychotic patients .... In a superficial sense, in that he can say he is in a psychiatric hospital because of his unacceptable and strange conduct, his insight is intact .... [Yet] he has absolutely no capacity to see himself as others see him."[2] Tom, Ernie, and Ed, the antisocial men we have encountered so far, cooperated during their initial evaluations. But all refused to accept the findings and to follow through with treatment, eventually demanding to be released against their doctors' advice. It is hard to convince an antisocial that something is wrong with him and even more difficult to persuade him to act accordingly. When the antisocial rejects efforts to help him and the law does not mandate treatment, there is no choice but to let him go.

Family members likewise may be difficult to convince that treatment is necessary. Many cling to the belief that their loved one simply has a few problems, just like anyone else, not the symptoms of a personality disorder. Some antisocials can deceive their families and friends for years, keeping their true selves hidden under a blanket of lies and empty promises. The charming, happy-go-lucky son just has a mean streak. The father is a good provider, despite his occasional disappearances and shady business dealings. As I find in my own work, some family members have the opposite reaction and are relieved to learn an ASP diagnosis. They are amazed by how well a description of ASP symptoms matches the characteristics displayed by their spouses, partners, parents, or children. Treatment often comes after repeated efforts by family members to change their loved ones' behavior through rewards, punishments, or emotional pleas, and they may embrace the diagnosis as the end to their frustrations and fears. In truth, it is only the beginning of a long and unpredictable process.

THE FIRST STEP

The first step in evaluating patients is to construct an accurate history through a careful interview. Because lab tests, x-rays, and brain scans have little, if any, diagnostic value—aside from their capacity to rule out other, organic problems—the patient's history is the most important basis for diagnosing ASP. A standard set of procedures and definitions provide guidelines for identifying antisocial personality and other mental disorders, but the diagnostic process ultimately is little more than an educated judgment call.[3] The same is true of many other medical diagnoses—all rely on some degree of experience, perception, and critical thinking.

The interview should begin with a sincere attempt to develop rapport with the patient. As a psychiatrist, I find that one useful strategy is to start by asking the patient about himself—what kind of work he does, where he goes to school, whether he is married or single, and so on. Questions should be asked in a manner that conveys genuine interest and does not make the patient feel that he is under interrogation. After rapport is established, the questions become more detailed and specific, circling in on the patient's problem and blending open-ended questions with others that easily can be answered "yes" or "no." By listening to the patient, the interviewer can observe how he moves from thought to thought and chooses to present information. The interview is important in each case, but its success obviously relies on the patient's willingness to cooperate and share truthful information.

The first goal of evaluation is to define the problem, the "chief complaint" that motivates a patient to seek treatment. Common chief complaints I've heard from people with ASP tend to center around their depression, substance abuse, anxiety, temper outbursts, and troubled relationships. I try to record the patient's own words, often statements like "My wife says she'll divorce me if I don't learn to control my temper." Questions about moods, behavior, thoughts and feelings, life circumstances, precipitating factors—anything that may uncover something about the patient's present state and possible illness—help shed light on the complaint.

In assessing an antisocial patient, family members and friends can become essential informants, able to fill in gaps in the patient's history or to interpret events as they actually happened, without the veneer of lies an antisocial may apply. Not surprising, one research study showed that family members are more accurate in describing their relatives' antisocial behavior than are the patients themselves.[4] Records from previous clinic or hospital visits can provide needed clues, including the impressions of other mental health professionals, and legal or educational documents may furnish additional pieces of the psychiatric jigsaw puzzle. Once confident that the completed picture presents an accurate view of a patient's past—and that the patient's problems are not caused by a medical condition—psychiatrists draw on the American Psychiatric Association's *Diagnostic and Statistical Manual of Mental Disorders, Fourth Edition, Text Revision* (DSM-IV-TR) criteria to help reach a judgment. More than one option may emerge. Many people with ASP are also alcoholic or clinically depressed and sometimes show traits of other personality disorders or mental illnesses. The psychiatrist records all of these diagnostic possibilities.

Early in our meeting, Paul described his recurring desire to masturbate before young girls, usually when motivated by drink. Although he did not seem to consider it a problem, his sexual conduct had sent him to the hospital in police custody and thus became the chief complaint in his case. Judging by his attitude, it is unlikely that he would have sought treatment for his bizarre sexual tastes on his own. Fortunately, he was forced into evaluation after committing a crime that is grounds for court-ordered therapy. Treatment for pedophilia is challenging and often unsuccessful, particularly when patients fail to see their actions as troublesome, and I suspected that Paul's problems were more than sexual—and that he could prove even more difficult to treat than other sex offenders. From the beginning, I sensed in Paul an underlying lack of concern for all sorts of social expectations. To determine his condition and prospects for the future, I would have to delve deep into his background.

PSYCHIATRIC HISTORY

One fundamental truth in psychiatry is that past behavior predicts future behavior, and that most problems severe enough to require treatment are not new to the individual. For that reason, assessing existing psychiatric records is a necessary early step in constructing a history. Mental health professionals pay special attention to any past diagnoses, beginning with those commonly identified during childhood, such as attention-deficit/hyperactivity disorder (ADHD) and conduct disorder. We also take note of past treatment, including medications, hospitalizations, and psychotherapy or counseling. Paging through these records can be like conferring with colleagues, as it reveals what other professionals have thought about the patient and his or her problems. It may help eliminate some diagnoses from consideration or even illuminate past mistakes in treatment. It also provides a chance to compare the official record with the patient's own account, highlighting important points where they differ or converge.

I asked Paul whether he had ever had mental or emotional problems and was mildly surprised by his candor. "I'm an alcoholic," he admitted, a relatively rare confession for antisocials and many other people with drinking problems. He had lost count of his hospitalizations for alcohol treatment but felt his chronic addiction was the root of many problems. His record showed 13 electroconvulsive or "shock" treatments during a hospital stay decades before, which implied a diagnosis of severe depression. But I found the most significant clue to his condition in a clinician's note: "[The patient] has demonstrated a long history of sociopathic behavior of the antisocial type. He has demonstrated poor judgment, lack of insight, irresponsibility, failure to profit from experience, failure to form any love relationships, and general irresponsibility." It confirmed that another psychiatrist had shared my initial hunch.

MEDICAL HISTORY

As physicians, psychiatrists are trained to assess the often complex interplay between physical and mental health, and—as with any medical diagnosis—understanding a patient's history of illness, surgical procedures, and medical treatment is vitally important. Use of alcohol, prescription medications, illicit drugs, and cigarette smoking warrant specific questions due to their potential for significant physical and psychological effects. All this information helps rule out some diagnostic possibilities and even suggests lifestyle modifications that can affect symptoms—for instance, reducing the intake of caffeine or other stimulants to counter anxiety.

When looking for evidence of ASP, interviewers ask about traumatic injuries and other phenomena that can suggest a reckless lifestyle. Many antisocials will have a history of head injury or motor vehicle and other accidents. Because ASP increases the risk of acquiring HIV and other sexually transmitted diseases, we inquire about them as well. A patient's ability to comply with treatment for any illness also can reveal details about his personality. For example, antisocials are well known for their tendency to leave hospitals against medical advice.[5]

Paul's alcoholism had had a profound impact on his physical and emotional health. Years earlier, he had developed alcohol-induced gastritis. He reported frequent blackouts and hallucinations when he went for more than a few days without a drink, claiming to see large spiders and snakes that quickly drove him back to whiskey. Alcoholic seizures sometimes plagued him, and he told of waking up to dry heaves caused by drinking and poor diet. Many years before, he had crashed his car into a culvert while drunk, and the injuries eventually required surgery to replace his right hip joint. In addition to alcohol, he had abused marijuana, amphetamines, and prescription pain killers. He had emphysema, but continued to chain smoke despite this and other health problems, including a bout with bladder cancer.

FAMILY HISTORY

Whether due to genetics, environment, or a combination of both, ASP passes from generation to generation in some families—families that also may be plagued with depression, alcoholism, drug addiction, ADHD, and other disorders. Information about the emotional and psychiatric health of parents, grandparents, aunts, uncles, and other relatives can help identify risk factors linked to heredity or home environment and can suggest possible diagnoses. Because a disproportionate percentage of antisocials are adoptees, many will be unfamiliar with their biological background.[6] Other patients may know little about their family history and are unable to cite any specific psychiatric diagnoses, yet they can describe a family member's drinking habits, bad temper, or long-term joblessness, thus providing valuable diagnostic clues.

Paul could offer little information about his family's mental health history. He was the only child of two working parents who seemed to enjoy a healthy and relatively happy marriage. His father was a baker, his mother a waitress in a local diner. In a tone that betrayed considerable hostility, he described his mother as "high strung" (considering what I later learned of his early behavior, Paul probably caused much of her distress). In contrast, Paul remembered his father as good-hearted and easy-going, always ready to bail his son out of difficult situations. By Paul's account, neither parent showed signs of serious mental illness, and he could report next to nothing about his grandparents, aunts, or uncles.

PERSONAL AND SOCIAL HISTORY

The details that indicate ASP tend to emerge as one asks a patient about the events of his life, from developmental milestones to criminal violations. When ASP is suspected based on the patient's chief complaint, the interviewer must address common problem areas for antisocials, most notably the symptoms described in the previous chapter. Collecting a broad range of evidence helps narrow the diagnostic possibilities, either supporting or contradicting the clinician's early hunches. Questions become focused and personal, probing for information that the patient may be unable or unwilling to provide.

The inquiry begins with anything the patient has been told about his birth, including difficulties with his delivery, and continues through early development and childhood problems like bedwetting—areas in which antisocials are likely to have had trouble.[7] The significance of bedwetting remains unclear, but it may reflect a lag in brain or central nervous system development, a problem linked to learning disorders and ADHD. Here again, psychiatric and medical records or accounts from informants may provide facts that the patient cannot.

The interviewer also explores early family life, including details about the home, the community, and any history of abuse. Educational background and troubles at school can yield significant clues, as can a sexual history that notes when the patient became sexually active, frequency of sexual relations, and sexual orientation. Major areas in which symptoms of ASP tend to emerge—work, relationships, military service, brushes with the law—are explored through the patient interview plus details from family members, friends, and official records. It is important to identify the number and type of jobs patients have held, periods of unemployment, relations with co-workers, and trouble complying with job requirements. Questions about marriage and relationships trace how they were initiated, what the mental status of partners has been, and whether domestic abuse occurred. Reports of military service history, criminal behavior, arrests, convictions, and incarceration can be compared with official documents when available.

Living arrangements, finances, and children are additional aspects of the personal history that help fill out the overall image of the patient's life, especially when ASP is a possibility. Frequency of moves, homelessness, and home ownership enter the picture, as do stability of income, credit history, and receipt of public assistance. If a patient has children, their number, ages, and health status are noted, along with whether the patient plays an active parental role. Further questions ask about abuse and neglect, and about whether the patient, if male, could have fathered additional children of whom he is unaware.

My suspicions about Paul and the source of his troubles guided our interview into areas where ASP symptoms tend to emerge. He willingly cooperated, speaking freely about his past. I was able to compare some of his claims with existing records and accepted others at face value. Whether true or not, the way Paul described his past told almost as much about his personality as did the content of his words.

Paul's birth was hard on his mother—a breech delivery after an extended labor. A nervous child, he routinely wet the bed until age eight, chewed his fingernails, and was plagued by nightmares, including one of a giant ball always rolling after him. He grew up in a small town, and his parents' jobs kept them outside the home, although never very far away. Paul told me he enjoyed his youthful independence and cultivated a rebellious streak that made for frequent trouble with parents, teachers, and just about any adult. He hated being told what to do, and the simplest instructions would inspire him to pursue the exact opposite. His interest in sex emerged unusually early. He claimed to have had intercourse at age eight, with an older neighbor girl who carefully coached him. Another early memory involved a girl—perhaps the same neighbor—removing his pants and beating his penis with a stick. He later began window peeping (which he denied having continued as an adult) and exposing himself to girls. His alcohol use also started while young and, by age 14, he was drinking at every opportunity, seldom stopping short of intoxication.

Not surprisingly, Paul cared little for education and dropped out of high school to join the Army, having tired of his hometown, his parents, and his persistent failures. Rigid military discipline ran contrary to his character, but he managed to complete a two-year enlistment without any major problems, and even completed a high school equivalency course. Once out of the Army, he dated a young woman who resisted his sexual advances and, after three weeks, he married her to get what he wanted. But even after the wedding, they remained sexually incompatible: He wanted sex during the day, she insisted on waiting until evening, and the situation soon degenerated into constant bickering. After giving birth to the first of their two sons, she found intercourse painful and began to refuse his requests for sex. He had begun pursuing other sexual outlets within weeks after their wedding and felt no regret about his infidelity. In fact, he boasted that during those days he could have sex with his pick of women.

When I asked Paul about his work history, he described a past notable even by antisocial standards, claiming to have held as many as 100 full-time jobs, the longest for 12 years. Records showed that this job—on an airplane assembly line—had really lasted for only five years, but it made little difference in his overall pattern of instability.

His deplorable work history started soon after he left the Army. He drifted from job to job, quitting once he tired of a particular position, usually with no alternative in sight. If he didn't quit, he was fired, often for drunkenness or absenteeism. Money was tight while he was living with his wife and sons, but never scarce enough to threaten his drinking, even if it meant that the boys had to go unfed. His wife left him after six years of marriage, taking the children with her, although the two of them never divorced. Paul did little to support his sons while they were growing up and attempted to justify his neglect by saying that they made him nervous. Both boys went on to experience their own troubles, wrestling with learning disabilities, behavior problems, drug use, and occasional arrests.

After the breakup of his family, Paul lived in "too many towns to count," sometimes moving "for the hell of it." He had relocated eight times in the decade before I evaluated him, finally settling when he inherited his parents' house. His failing health slowed him down, and he had been living on disability and a small veteran's pension since cancer surgery four years before. By his own account, he had been arrested "150 times, easy," mostly on minor charges related to alcohol, but also for four felonies. Despite his record, some of which I was able to confirm, he had never spent more than six months in jail. He had little interest in socializing, although he claimed to be a jovial drunk who offered to buy rounds at the neighborhood bar. Of people in general, he said he could "take them or leave them." He continued to resist authority in even the most trivial ways, refusing to wear a seat belt while driving simply because it was the law.

Paul's account of his life confirmed my initial suspicions. The pattern of antisocial behavior observed during his hospitalization years before had continued, and Paul's problem with exhibitionism seemed rooted in a deep-seated personality disturbance. Despite his near textbook depiction of an antisocial lifestyle, there remained a few necessary steps before I could make a diagnosis. But with Paul's history in mind, I knew I was approaching a conclusion.

PSYCHOLOGICAL TESTS AND OTHER CLUES

While collecting essential background information, mental health professionals train their attention on patients' appearance, habits, and demeanor, noting any peculiarities in dress, attitude, or speaking style. Patients may speak with unusual speed or determination, may avoid eye contact, or may assume a defensive tone—all characteristics that shed light on their personalities and color what they say. Their orientation to time, place, and person; ability to reason; and memory can be assessed informally in a mental status examination (MSE). The MSE can help show whether a patient suffers from delusions or has significant intellectual impairments. It usually involves asking patients to remember certain words, perform simple calculations, and interpret common proverbs. Although abnormal responses or poor cognitive performance alone do not rule out ASP, they may give important clues to other mental illnesses or to medical disorders that can cause or contribute to antisocial behavior.

I've already noted some of the qualities Paul unwittingly displayed during our interview, including the nervous cues that betrayed his need for a drink. When he talked about himself, however, his agitation gave way to a relaxed frankness. He seemed to have no qualms about relating the events of his past, sometimes bragging about his experiences, no matter how unsavory. His apparent comfort with his deviant behavior, the ease with which he discussed breaking every rule, was consistent with ASP. Despite the long-term effects of his alcoholism, his lack of concern for himself or anyone else, and his pattern of bad decisions, I thought Paul was reasonably intelligent. He seemed wholly able to perceive reality, and I saw little evidence of a mental illness that would cloud his ability to judge right from wrong.

Had I needed additional information, I might have administered a range of psychological tests to explore Paul's thinking patterns and assess his intellectual capacity. These tests can be especially helpful when patients refuse to permit interviews with relatives or have no other informants. In these cases, the tests can provide crucial bits of information that supplement the patient's own words.

Although I don't request this test very often with my antisocial patients, the Minnesota Multiphasic Personality Inventory (MMPI) is clearly one of the most frequently used personality measures. Its 556 true-false questions assess nine pathological dimensions and yield a broad profile of personality functioning. One of the dimensions is called *psychopathic deviance*—a term that dates to early versions of the MMPI.[8] The MMPI also measures truthfulness of responses with questions that tend to be answered a certain way only when the patient is trying to make himself look better—for instance, queries about mild and common misbehaviors that most people readily admit.

As mentioned in Chapter 2, the Psychopathy Checklist–Revised (PCL-R) was developed by psychologist Robert Hare to assess the presence and severity of psychopathic traits, such as glibness, callousness, and lack of remorse. There is little reason to obtain a PCL-R in routine evaluations of antisocial patients, but it may be extremely valuable in certain research or prison settings because it appears to predict reoffending and parole violations, which are of particular relevance to correctional staff.[9]

Projective tests thought to tap the patient's unconscious mental processes are sometimes used. The best known is the *Rorschach*, or ink blot test, which consists of 10 standard (and meaningless) images patients are asked to interpret.[10] Shown a particular image, one patient may see a butterfly where another sees two men dancing. Based on these perceptions, the psychologist conducting the test attempts to draw conclusions about the patient's personality. Antisocials, for example, may report seeing things that reflect their preoccupations, perhaps scenes involving domination, thievery, or violence.

Tests of intelligence and educational achievement can also provide useful information, although no particular result indicates ASP. The revised Wechsler Adult Intelligence Scale is perhaps the most commonly used test of intelligence, but there are many from which to choose. Research shows that juvenile delinquents and criminals (groups that overlap with ASP) have significantly lower IQs than controls, generally on the order of around 10 points, and are also more likely to show evidence of learning disabilities.[11] To some experts, these findings provide circumstantial evidence that antisocial behavior results from a more generalized brain disorder. To others, they help explain the poor academic achievement, bad work records, and low economic status of many antisocials.

In his book *Inside the Criminal Mind*, Stanton E. Samenow dismisses any link between learning disabilities and criminal behavior, describing a typically antisocial response to education: "Many criminals who appear learning disabled are highly capable of learning but choose not to do so .... They may not learn what parents and teachers want them to learn."[12] Nonetheless, educational tests sometimes help pinpoint specific deficits that may inhibit a person's school or job performance, and identifying specific learning disabilities might help explain long-term problems or provide goals for therapy.

Other scales and tests can be used to measure the impact of particular mental health or behavioral problems, and these are selected at the psychiatrist's discretion based on what the patient reveals about his life and circumstances.[13] The Beck Depression Inventory can be helpful in assessing those who indicate a history of sadness, apathy, or suicidal behavior, whereas the Michigan Assessment and Screening Test can be used to measure a patient's dependence on alcohol. The

Buss-Durkee Inventory likewise can help assess aggressive tendencies, whereas the Barratt Impulsiveness Scale can help assess the person's potential for impulsive acting-out. Paul's relationship with alcohol was fairly well established, as was his history of depression and aggression. In his case, psychological tests were unnecessary, although I have sometimes found them helpful in assessing younger patients with shorter histories or others with less detailed records.

There are no medical tests for ASP, but specific laboratory tests may be prompted by the patient's medical history, such as tests for sexually transmitted diseases or tests to assess liver function in alcoholic patients. A complete evaluation of the patient generally includes a physical examination. Evidence of injury from fights or accidents, past knife or gunshot wounds, scars from injuries that may have been self-inflicted, or even evidence of nail biting are common among antisocials.[14] Physical signs of alcohol or drug abuse may be present, for example, an enlarged liver or track marks from repeated intravenous drug injections.

Tattoos have traditionally been considered markers of ASP because—at least in the past—they were so common in antisocials, especially those marked by violence or aggression.[15] As tattoos have become increasingly faddish among today's youth, they are no longer the specific markers they once were, and some feel they are no longer suggestive of ASP. Yet, they still have a power to suggest nonconformity, and, as we have seen, many men portrayed in this book have tattoos. Some, like Tom, have crude do-it-yourself tattoos acquired in prison. Others sport elaborate designs celebrating relationships or gang affiliations.

Paul showed some of these signs when I examined him, none of which surprised me in light of his medical history. The injuries sustained in his car accident years before continued to plague him. He walked with a pronounced limp, his right leg about two inches shorter than his left. His voice was deep and rough from years of smoking, and he had a vicious dry cough. His body bore the marks of countless minor injuries, scars that betrayed a history of bar fights and intoxication-related clumsiness.

THE DIFFERENTIAL DIAGNOSIS

When the history has been pieced together, the time comes to consider potential explanations for the patient's chief complaint and current problems, a process that results in the *differential diagnosis*, a set of possibilities ranked from most to least probable. When ASP makes the list, it opens up new avenues of investigation, because an array of other disorders must be ruled out before it can be diagnosed. Consider, for example, a patient with a violent temper. Some rare forms of epilepsy, such as temporal lobe epilepsy (TLE), cause random outbursts of violence not triggered by a particular stress or situation. A person with TLE may enter a trancelike state during these episodes and later be unable to recall what happened. Although some antisocials may claim to forget their violent or criminal behaviors—not uncommon in prisoners—the pattern that emerges in legitimate TLE cases is very different from that usually seen in ASP. Assessment with special electroencephalographic (EEG) tracings can help pin down the diagnosis of epilepsy.

Tumors, strokes, and traumatic injuries can cause brain damage that leads to personality changes. Such conditions were once called *organic personality disorders*, but *DSM-IV-TR* now uses the straightforward term *personality change resulting from a general medical condition*. With these disorders, the patient's underlying temperament commonly emerges in an exaggerated form, but irritability, angry outbursts, and low tolerance for frustration are also common. Significant brain injuries usually can be visualized with scans using magnetic resonance imaging (MRI) or computed tomography (CT), but subtle injuries may escape detection. Information from the patient's history also helps eliminate illness or injury as causes of uncharacteristic violence or dark moods. Personality changes in people with brain injuries are notable for their relatively recent appearance, and they are unlikely to have a history of childhood delinquency. The antisocial, of course, has a lifelong tendency toward bad behavior, and it is this consistency, rather than any sudden change, that characterizes ASP.

Antisocial personality must also be distinguished from bipolar (manic-depressive) disorder and schizophrenia. These conditions have characteristic patterns and symptoms that help in separating them from ASP. For example, schizophrenia leads to delusional thinking and frightening hallucinations, combined with profound personality changes that affect emotions and motivational drive. Bipolar disorder leads to wild mood swings with sustained highs and lows. In routine practice, it generally isn't too difficult to separate ASP from these conditions, but occasional patients appear to have *both* disorders. In my work as a prison consultant, I have seen many offenders over the years with clear-cut schizophrenia, but who also appear to have been severely antisocial before they developed their psychotic illness. I find these patients particularly menacing because they not only have a lack of conscience stemming from their ASP, but sometimes act in response to their delusions.

Once these conditions have been ruled out, the psychiatrist should identify and diagnose any additional disorders that may be present, such as depression, an anxiety disorder, an addiction, pathological gambling, or a psychosexual disturbance. In truth, it may have been one of these coexisting disorders that was the driving force that led the person to seek help, not the ASP. It is essential to diagnose coexisting disorders because some have specific treatments, as will be discussed later in this book. Antisocials with depression may benefit from antidepressant medication, for instance, whereas those with drug or alcohol addictions may need a rehabilitation program. Those with ADHD might benefit from stimulant medication to improve their attention and behavior, although these medications are usually not an option for the antisocial whose life has been complicated by addiction, because of their abuse potential. Relationship counseling can help antisocials and their partners, and the support that family members can offer makes the efforts to mend broken ties an important part of therapy. These options are explored further in Chapter 7.

An EEG tracing of Paul's brain waves appeared mildly abnormal but was not compatible with a diagnosis of epilepsy. Besides, although Paul showed signs of aggression tempered by age and disability, his problem was not sporadic violence but rather exhibitionism and other blatant violations of social norms. Routine laboratory tests and a physical examination helped rule out brain injury and other medical conditions as the cause of his behavior. Similarly, Paul showed no evidence of schizophrenia or bipolar disorder. He no doubt struggled with depression and alcoholism, and readily conceded the latter, which was the only thing he truly seemed to regret about his life. Repeated attempts to stop drinking—Alcoholics Anonymous, hospital programs, and other efforts—had produced only short-term success, and, although I would recommend alcohol treatment, I had little hope that it would work. Paul's other immediate problem was his abnormal sexual interest in young girls, but I likewise doubted he would benefit from a treatment program for sex offenders.

MAKING THE DIAGNOSIS

By this point, I had assembled the clues. My interview with Paul was complete. I had collected and reviewed his medical, legal, and educational records. The necessary examinations and tests were finished, and I had considered a range of alternative diagnoses. In this case, as in all others, I drew on training and experience to make the diagnosis, which could have profound implications for the patient.

Skeptics may downplay the significance of psychiatric diagnoses, ASP included, and some of their criticisms are understandable, considering that psychiatry—like other branches of medicine—relies on educated judgments and skills that vary from person to person. Nevertheless, a psychiatric diagnosis is not simply a label, a self-fulfilling prophesy, or even, as some suggest, an excuse for a person's flaws. Rather, it carries several important functions and can help guide a troubled patient toward a more fulfilling life.

First, a psychiatric diagnosis helps to clarify the complex clinical phenomena characteristic of mental illness. Faced with a broad and blurred range of emotional, cognitive, and behavioral abnormalities that can manifest themselves in varied ways, psychiatry has developed diagnostic categories to impose a modicum of order on this chaos. In doing so, it makes mental illnesses easier to understand for professionals in training, patients, and the families and friends of people with psychiatric disorders, and it facilitates communication between clinicians. When I give a patient's symptoms a specific description, such as ASP, this concise statement enables health professionals who later study the patient's records to draw tentative conclusions about the clinical picture. Basically, the *DSM* categories are a form of professional shorthand.

Psychiatric diagnoses also help predict what lies ahead for a patient. Like many other psychiatric disorders, ASP is associated with a characteristic course and outcome. The diagnosis alerts the patient's caregivers to potential problems and complications that may arise. The diagnosis can also serve as a wake-up call to patients and may spur them to seek help.

Finally, diagnoses are important to psychiatric researchers, helping them assemble groups of persons with similar symptoms and problems. Researchers are thus better able to investigate risk factors that may be associated with different disorders, as well as to study possible treatments. The ultimate goal of this research is to isolate the causes of disorders like ASP and to develop more specific and effective treatments.

Readers should resist the temptation to diagnose themselves or others with ASP after learning about the disorder here or elsewhere. Nonetheless, I have provided a list of questions to offer a rough guideline of queries that psychiatrists and other mental health professionals may use to explore the possibility of ASP. The questions are not part of any formal questionnaire, do not follow any particular order, and have no special meaning apart from the fact that they represent the types of problems, behaviors, and attitudes common to antisocials.

1. Do you have a short fuse and a hair-trigger temper?
2. When in trouble, do you blame others?
3. Have you had trouble keeping a job?
4. Have you ever quit a job out of anger without another one to go to?
5. Do you get into frequent fights?
6. Have you ever physically or verbally hurt your spouse?
7. Have you ever not paid child support required by law?
8. Have you ever failed to follow through on financial obligations?
9. Have you ever vandalized or destroyed property?
10. Have you ever pursued an illegal occupation like selling drugs or prostituting yourself?
11. Have you ever harassed or stalked others?
12. As a child, did you ever skip school?
13. Have you ever been cruel to small animals, like cats or dogs?
14. Have you ever moved to a new location without having a job lined up?
15. Have you ever been homeless or lacked a fixed address?

16. Have you ever wandered around the country without any clear goal in mind about where you were going?
17. Have you ever stolen or burglarized?
18. If you were in the military, did you ever go absent without leave (AWOL)?
19. If you have a tattoo, does it have a violent or gang associated theme?
20. Have you ever used an alias or gone by another name?
21. Do you tend to be impulsive and make decisions without reflection?
22. Have you ever run a "scam" or tried to con others?
23. Have you ever lied to obtain sexual favors from another?
24. Were you ever suspended or expelled from school because of your behavior?
25. As a child, did you ever set fires?
26. Have you ever thought about harming or killing someone?
27. Do you tend to disregard laws that you don't like, such as those against speeding?
28. Have you ever beaten or abused your children?
29. Are you sexually promiscuous?
30. Did you ever use a weapon in a fight as a child?
31. Did you engage in sexual activity before most of your peers did?
32. Have you ever abused alcohol or other drugs?
33. Have you ever mugged anyone?
34. Have you been fired from jobs because of personality problems?
35. As a child, did you ever lie to authority figures, like parents, teachers, or supervisors?
36. Have you ever been arrested or convicted of a felony?
37. Was your behavior incorrigible as a youngster?
38. Did you ever have to go to a reform school or detention center as a juvenile?

39. Have you ever been jailed or imprisoned?

40. Have you ever squandered money on personal items rather than buying necessities for your family?

41. Are you relatively unconcerned about having hurt or mistreated others?

42. Did you ever run away from home as a child?

43. Were you ever adopted or placed in foster care as a child?

44. Have you ever snatched a purse or picked someone's pocket?

45. Did you ever move to avoid the authorities?

46. Have you ever forged someone else's name on a document, like a check?

47. Have you been married and divorced more than twice?

48. Do you feel that you are better than everyone else and therefore above the law?

49. Do you feel that the world owes you a living?

50. Have you ever forced someone to have sexual relations with you?

THE RESULT

I diagnosed Paul as antisocial based on his history, demeanor, and lack of any other medical or psychiatric illness that could explain his troubles. Although I noted additional diagnoses of depression, alcoholism, and sexual deviance (exhibitionism), his pattern of remorseless misbehavior indicated that the root of his problems was a personality disorder, a consistent inability to adapt to the expectations that most of us effortlessly embrace. I never saw Paul after completing his evaluation, but I later found that he had been convicted of exposing himself to the girl and was ordered to complete counseling for his alcoholism and sexual problems. As is usually the case, Paul's

ASP was not addressed by the courts, having gone unattended since it was first suggested in his psychiatric records decades before. He had lived with ASP for many years and, considering his failing health and the tendency for antisocials of his age to gradually abandon their more destructive behaviors, his case seemed far less threatening than many others, despite his habit of exposing himself and committing other troublesome acts.

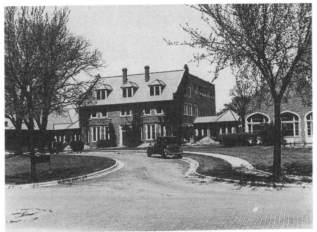

The men in the Black's study were hospitalized at the University of Iowa Psychiatric Hospital (formerly Psychopathic Hospital) in Iowa City. This photo dates from the 1930s (Courtesy of the University of Iowa).

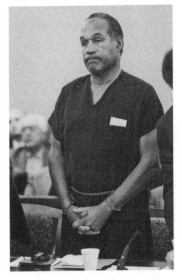

O.J. Simpson, former football star and actor who many believe killed his wife Nicole, now sits in a Nevada prison (Getty Images).

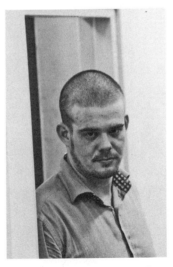

Joran van der Sloot, implicated in the disappearance of college student Natalee Holloway on Aruba, was convicted of murdering a Peruvian woman in 2010 (Getty Images).

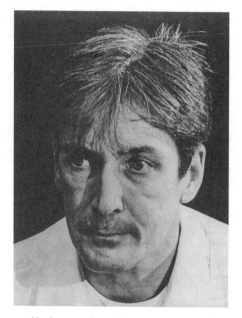

Gary Gilmore, executed by firing squad in Utah in 1977, was famously quoted to say "Let's do it" (Getty Images).

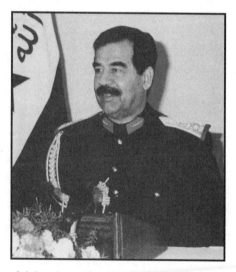

Saddam Hussein ruled through a combination of ruthlessness and cruelty. He was toppled from power in the Iraq War in 2003. He was later executed by hanging (Getty Images).

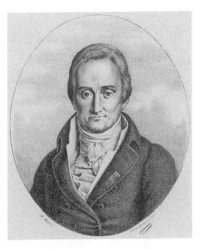

Phillipe Pinel, leader of the French Revolution and founding father of modern psychiatry, used the term *manie sans délire* to describe antisocial behavior.

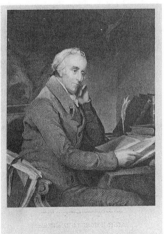

Benjamin Rush, a physician who signed the Declaration of Independence and founded what later became the American Psychiatric Association, provided one of the first descriptions of antisocial behavior (Courtesy of the University of Pennsylvania).

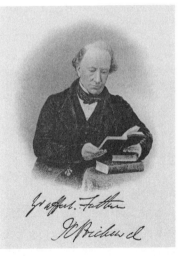

British physician James Prichard coined the term "moral insanity" in 1835.

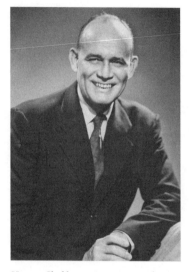

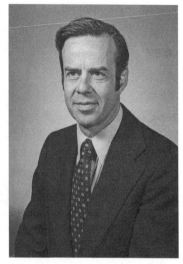

Hervey Cleckly, an American psychiatrist, wrote the bestselling book *The Mask of Sanity*, but is better known for co-authoring *The Three Faces of Eve* (with Corbett Thigpen) (Getty Images).

Robert Spitzer, a Columbia University psychiatrist, led the charge to develop criteria-based diagnoses in DSM-III (Courtesy of Robert Spitzer).

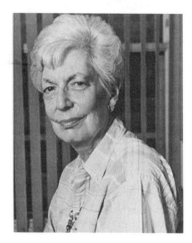

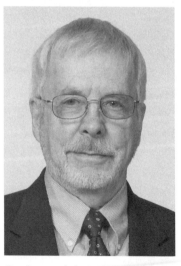

Lee Robins, a sociologist at Washington University, was responsible for inspiring the ASP criteria in DSM-III.

Canadian psychologist Robert Hare has championed the notion of psychopathy as distinct from ASP.

Chapter 5

Divergent Paths

The Natural History of
Antisocial Personality Disorder

FORETELLING THE FUTURE

The bleak picture of antisocial personality disorder (ASP) emerges in lives like Paul's, whom we met in Chapter 4. Rebellious boys who torment their parents with pathological defiance grow into troubled adults who lie, commit crimes, take up alcohol or drugs, and beat their spouses—or worse. None of the stories I have shared thus far has a happy ending, and this is usually the case with ASP. The diagnosis predicts what may be in store for patients and might help persuade them to seek treatment or, at the very least, to understand that they have a problem. Predictions have their limits, of course, and patients with ASP may take similar routes to different destinations.

Much of my work with antisocials—including the research on which this book is based—involves an effort to understand where this disorder leads those whom it affects. I am not alone in attempting to chart the natural history of ASP, but all the existing research leaves us still looking for answers. Some may wonder why we care what happens to men who seem capable of perceiving reality and making decisions but who consistently choose to do the wrong things. We care because ASP is a serious problem, with a much greater impact than is generally recognized. We also care because knowing what happens to antisocials over time might uncover clues to assist others who struggle with the disorder. Antisocial personality disorder research seeks to identify risk factors and predictors of outcome, information that may help us find ways to treat—or even to prevent—the disorder. But, at present, our knowledge of predictors makes us painfully aware of our limited capacity to intervene.

Although existing research may not say as much as we might like about the course of ASP, it permits some general observations. The most basic fact about the disorder's progression is the link between conduct problems in childhood and adult misbehavior, which gives this book its title. Most troubled children do not become antisocial adults, but those who do often stand apart early in life. Not surprisingly, the most difficult kids are most likely to keep acting out as they grow older, but even those who show the earliest and worst symptoms can improve. This chapter details research on how ASP unfolds over the course of a patient's life. It includes the stories of two men whose lives bear the startling similarities found across cases of ASP, but whose stories also show how this disorder can have more than one outcome.

LIVES IN COMMON

James Baker had no true memory of his birth parents. He was only two when they divorced, sending him and his two older brothers to an orphanage. None of them had any further contact with their parents, who Jim later described in derogatory terms based on what he had been told: His father was a "vagabond," his mother a "religious fanatic." The orphanage terrified the young boy and left him with recollections of being locked in closets or being made to lie on the stone floor when he refused to take a nap. Regularly punished for wetting his bed, he experienced the taunts and abuse of older boys and remained an outsider in a lonely world of abandoned children. After placement in three different foster homes, Jim was adopted by an older couple who seemed to see past his record of behavior problems. He would later describe his adoptive mother as a "nagging, overbearing, authoritarian, old-maid schoolteacher type" with a knack for vicious scolding. He remembered her husband as gentle and calm but "half-drunk all the time."

In another place, at about the same time, Doug Baughman was trying his parents' patience with lies and temper tantrums set off by the simplest requests. He loathed authority of any kind, ignoring household chores and homework assignments. As he grew older, Doug became an expert shoplifter and also began burglarizing neighborhood homes and cars for anything that caught his eye or could be sold. Despite his 125 IQ, he was a failure at school, flunking nearly every course, insulting his teachers, and disrupting class with abrasive remarks. His academic career ended in high school with a suspension for smoking on school grounds, which he took as an opportunity to drop out for good.

Like Doug, Jim had trouble with school. From the beginning, it had brought back the torments of the orphanage, and the loud, disruptive boy often was set apart from others as punishment for his misbehavior. He longed for friendship but alienated himself with clownish pranks and other clumsy grabs for attention. Eventually, he fell in with a gang known for shoplifting and burglary and was glad to have found a sense of belonging after years of bouncing from place to place. He managed to stay in school and progress through the grades until he finally dropped out during his senior year of high school. He further dismayed his parents by leaving home for days at a time, seeming to share his biological father's affinity for aimless wandering. At age 17, he joined the Marines and served 18 months in Korea, learning to handle military discipline and earning the nickname "Dirty Jim" for his combat prowess.

Doug's teenage years were even more turbulent. By age 18, he had acquired a record of psychiatric hospitalizations, the first after he was caught stealing cigarettes from a store where he worked. The owner immediately fired him and contacted the police. In response, Doug slashed his own left arm with a scalpel stolen days earlier from a physician's car. He spent a few days in the hospital for observation but was released by psychiatrists who found no evidence of clinical depression. He returned to the hospital three months later at his parents' request. Breaking into cars was bad enough, but his mother was more disturbed by Doug's raid on the family Christmas fund. Several neighborhood girls also recognized Doug as the boy spotted peeping through their bedroom windows.

His parents, following the thinking of the day, hoped that psychiatrists could identify a buried psychological cause for his behavior, perhaps something they had done wrong that was not beyond remedy. Doug had little interest in discussing his delinquency and claimed his problem was brief bouts of depression that resulted from such snubs as a girl's refusal to dance with him. His doctors surmised that Doug felt rejected by his parents, overlooked in favor of his siblings, and suggested that he be placed in a boarding school or foster home. Instead, his parents took him back. Months later, he overdosed on his mother's tranquilizers and cut both forearms with a razor blade. Affirming their earlier assessment, the doctors interpreted Doug's behavior as a manipulative effort to get out of the house and back to the hospital. He stayed for three months, then was transferred to the state reformatory until he was old enough to provide for himself. At age 18, he was released and moved to Baltimore, where he met up with a friend and hoped to make a fresh start.

BEGINNINGS

As the parents of many antisocials would attest, the behaviors that grow into full-fledged ASP begin early, often before children enter school. Boys who later develop the disorder usually have behavior problems by ages 8–10, although their mothers may recall serious troubles much earlier. In girls, symptoms may not emerge until puberty. A child who makes it to age 15 without exhibiting such behaviors will never develop ASP, according to sociologist Lee Robins, who asserts that "adult antisocial behavior virtually requires childhood antisocial behavior." The American Psychiatric Association's *Diagnostic and Statistical Manual of Mental Disorders, Fourth Edition, Text Revision* (*DSM-IV-TR*) definition of ASP includes a history of *conduct disorder*—the term for persistent childhood behavior problems—as one criterion for the diagnosis.[1] Because misbehavior is common in children, early troubles may be overlooked or explained away as short-term problems, while its true significance goes unrecognized.

Sheldon and Eleanor Glueck, working at Harvard Law School in the 1940s and 1950s, were among the first to observe that some adults who commit antisocial acts are continuing a pattern of behavioral problems established in childhood. Although innovative and groundbreaking, their work was largely ignored because the husband and wife team were considered academic outcasts. The Gluecks had followed 500 boys between the ages of 10 and 17 judged "officially delinquent" by the Massachusetts correctional system. The boys were studied intensively and contacted for follow-up interviews at ages 25, 32, and 45. The best-known result of this research, the Gluecks' book *Unraveling Juvenile Delinquency*, was published in 1950, but many of its observations continue to hold up today.[2] In the 1990s, psychologists Robert Sampson and John Laub conducted a computer-aided reanalysis of the Gluecks' study, confirming its original findings.[3] Severe antisocial behavior in childhood—problems serious enough to constitute delinquency in the eyes of the law—remained strongly linked to adult crime and deviance. Arrests between ages 17 and 32 were three to four times more likely to occur among men who had been delinquent boys than in their nondelinquent peers. Childhood antisocial behavior also predicted educational achievement, economic status, employment, and family life when delinquent boys grew up. Sampson and Laub concluded that the Gluecks' research showed "a stable tendency toward criminality and other troublesome behavior.... From this viewpoint, the varied outcomes correlated with childhood behavior are all expressions of the same underlying trait or propensity."[4]

In the 1950s—the time when Jim and Doug were showing their first signs of trouble—Lee Robins conducted a seminal study that revealed much of what we know about the natural history of ASP.

Her book, *Deviant Children Grown Up*, echoed the Gluecks' findings, which she cites in her book, this time linking serious juvenile delinquency with ASP in adulthood.[5] Hoping to discover which troubled children became antisocial adults, Robins and her research team searched for 524 subjects who had been counseled at a child guidance clinic between 1922 and 1932. The children averaged 13 years of age when seen at the clinic, nearly three-quarters were boys, and most were referred there directly from juvenile court. Theft charges were the most common cause for being sent to the clinic, followed by incorrigibility (defiance of parental rules, staying out late, refusing to work or help at home), learning problems, sexual offenses, and running away from home.

It took several years and considerable ingenuity for Robins and her team, but they succeeded in locating 90% of the subjects, an average of 30 years after their clinic visits. The investigators gathered information anywhere they could, interviewing relatives; investigating court records and police logs; and poring over reports from schools, orphanages, and other institutions. Once found, nearly two-thirds of the subjects contacted agreed to follow-up interviews. In her book, Robins describes the challenges of the search and the small victories the researchers enjoyed:

> Some of the successful methods bear all the earmarks of a detective story.... One man's family was located but refused to give his address. In consternation, his sister said, "He has enough trouble raising his kids and dogs without being bothered by you." On the strength of this statement we called the local kennel club and asked how we might find a man who raised dogs. We were referred to the president of the local collie club, who remembered the name because our subject had recently placed an ad in the collie club newsletter. She gave us his address and we interviewed him.[6]

The good news, Robins learned, was that most subjects improved as they grew older and did not become antisocial adults. Those who continued to make trouble had an earlier onset of behavior problems and showed a greater variety of problems than the others. Their childhood behaviors were more severe, and their first arrests occurred at early ages. Robins observed that only those who showed at least six kinds of antisocial behavior and had four or more episodes of such behavior—or at least one episode serious enough to result in a court appearance—were later diagnosed as sociopathic personalities. In milder cases, behavior problems were eventually outgrown.

Although the work of the Gluecks and Robins show the continuity of misbehavior throughout the lives of some subjects, they indicate that most behaviorally disturbed children do *not* grow up to become antisocial. Terrie Moffitt, a psychologist at the Duke University Institute for Brain Sciences, suggests that only a small number of men—perhaps 5%—demonstrate highly stable patterns of extreme antisocial behavior, and she has described their disorder as *life-course-persistent.*[7] Most troubled kids, according to Moffitt, have a less severe *adolescence-limited* behavioral disorder linked to teenage peer pressure. These teenagers typically have little or no history of earlier antisocial behavior and will improve on their own, Moffitt says, accounting for the fact that most children diagnosed with conduct disorder do not develop adult ASP. Some antisocial behavior is normal in children, and Moffitt estimates that up to 60% of adolescent boys engage in some form of delinquency. But most shape up as they mature, their mild "crime careers" confined to their teenage years.

One factor that moderates the eventual outcome of childhood misbehavior is a child's degree of socialization—his or her tendency to form relationships and internalize social norms. The late Richard Jenkins, a noted child psychiatrist at the University of Iowa, and whom I knew in his later years, believed that the ability to develop group loyalty is crucial and marks a fundamental division among children with conduct disorder.[8] Socialized children, regardless of their behavior, form strong ties to a familiar group of friends, whereas undersocialized children tend to be loners. In a 10-year follow-up study, Jenkins and his colleagues found that socialized delinquents were less likely to have been convicted of crimes or imprisoned. These children conformed to group rules and developed delinquent behavior from peer group pressure, whereas those who continued to exhibit antisocial behavior did not form such a group identity.

Like Doug and Jim, boys who become antisocial men stand out from the crowd by virtue of their varied and persistent problems during childhood. They tend to defy authority and reject the rules before most of their peers do, and they maintain their pattern of behavior long after other troublesome kids have gone on to better things. As these boys grow up, things only get worse.

BAD BOYS GROWN UP

Having come to like the military, "Dirty Jim" availed himself of the many opportunities offered by his stint in Korea. He learned to drink as he had learned to fight—alongside fellow Marines who urged him on and cheered his prowess. He dabbled in the widely available narcotics and slept with prostitutes but, unlike most of his comrades-in-arms, he also had a brief sexual relationship with a fellow Marine. When his tour was over, he returned home to his old pattern of drifting from place to place, job to job, bar to bar, but soon met a young woman who encouraged him to enroll at a state college. Their relationship grew, and they married when she discovered she was pregnant. A second child followed, but after an ambitious start—at least by his standards—Jim sensed himself failing in his attempt at family life. He felt no particular closeness to his wife or children and had a deepening sense that the years since Korea had been wasted. Once again, he felt alone. Finally, compelled by his wife and his own dark feelings, he made his first trip to a psychiatrist.

Doug, on the other hand, was well versed in the psychiatric routine that had given him the chance to escape from home and make what he saw as a new life. Within weeks of his arrival in Baltimore, he met, briefly dated, and eloped with a young woman, despite the stern objections of her parents. Marriage did not dispel his old habits, however, and soon he resumed his petty burglaries and window peeping. A few months after the wedding, he bungled a raid on the auto dealership across the street from the apartment he shared with his wife. Unable to open the safe, he set the place on fire and was arrested and convicted of arson. He was sentenced to seven years at the Patuxent Institute, a therapeutic prison that featured intensive therapy for young offenders.[9] Prisoners had indeterminate sentences that kept them locked up until they improved, and cooperation was essential if one was to be released. Doug held a prison job, followed the rules, and attended therapy, perhaps aided by his teenage experiences with psychiatrists and institutions.

His restraint broke, however, when his wife sought a divorce, prompting him to slash his wrists in a fit of anger. But he soon recovered and was eventually released two years early for good behavior. Once he was back on the streets, his improvement proved short-lived. He was arrested for window peeping only a month later and was jailed for 30 days. A whirlwind romance followed his release, then a second marriage. After a series of brief, dead-end jobs, Doug settled into something he was good at—tending bar. Although never much of a drinker before, he developed a taste for alcohol and broke his boss's ban on drinking at work. Liquor became his crutch, erasing guilt for past mistakes and, he later claimed, quieting his violent fantasies involving young girls and gay men. Sex had become both a treasured vice and a torment for Doug. Less than a year after his wedding, he impregnated a married woman in a clandestine affair. At home, he could only reach orgasm during intercourse with his wife by describing to her his fantasies of sodomizing a neighbor girl. Since his stay in the Patuxent Institute, he had been haunted by homosexual urges, which he maintained were the result of being paid for sex with another man. Tempted by desires he feared—as well as by thoughts of burglary—he punished himself by slashing his left calf with a razor blade. Doug's wife demanded that he seek psychiatric help.

Also prompted by inner turmoil and his wife's pleading, Jim had seen a psychiatrist, who described his behavior as "individualistic … bordering on criminal" and noted his inability to form close attachments and his "promiscuous sexual life." He was referred to the psychiatric hospital at the University of Iowa, where he told his admitting physician about his lack of feeling for his family, his reliance on alcohol, and his troubles with work. He described powerful bouts of depression, the latest after failing a real estate examination that would have allowed him to work as an agent. Some of the symptoms he described—growing feelings of anxiety, trouble concentrating and remembering—indicated depression, but he denied having the sleep disturbance, weight loss, and lapses in sexual drive typically associated with the condition. Nonetheless, his thoughts of suicide, particularly his tentative plan to cut his wrists, showed how serious his state had become. He also confessed thoughts about murdering someone else, although he refused to say who.

Jim tried hard to gain insight into his own emotions, perhaps driven by his need to understand the depression into which he had collapsed. He admitted feeling different from others, failing where everyone else seemed to succeed. During therapy, he made statements like "If you have a brain and don't use it, you might as well be a bum" and "If I am so right and everything turns out wrong, then I must be wrong." The psychiatrist described Jim's tendency to intellectualize and added, "He feels that he is self-critical and perhaps looks too hard to find things in himself." His hospital stay lasted for three weeks and included interviews conducted under the influence of sodium amytal and the stimulant methedrine—a common technique at the time—but most of the psychiatric observations concerned his behavior on the ward. Despite Jim's professed desire to understand his problem, his doctor's discharge note described Jim's lack of cooperation and limited understanding. He was "unrealistic, selfish, had not profited from past experiences and used denial.... He expected a magical cure from the hospital." The diagnosis was "sociopathic personality, antisocial reaction," the term *reaction* denoting the then-common belief in psychiatry that abnormal emotions were the expression of hidden conflicts. His prognosis was listed as poor, and no treatments were recommended.

Five years later, Jim returned to the hospital at age 32. His antisocial behavior had continued, and his alcoholism had become chronic. The wife who had once said she could not imagine leaving him had been granted a divorce. Jim's work was sporadic, and he was unable to make court-ordered alimony and child support payments. He wrote to one of the doctors seeking help: "At the present I am unemployed.... I feel I am unable to successfully work for anyone despite my endeavors. My personality and emotions are too deeply seated, as you probably know. I would still like to try to improve my stability, which is sadly lacking." Upon his return to treatment, he seemed more open and honest, and admitted to being a "subtle manipulator" who had cheated on his wife throughout their marriage in affairs with both women and men. He was involved in the antique trade, where he had developed a hustler's reputation for rapid buying and selling.

The doctor described Jim's attitude as "cocky and superior," hardly conducive to psychiatric treatment. At one point, asked what he hoped to accomplish in therapy, Jim remarked, "Don't try to play cat-and-mouse with me and I won't try to play cat-and-mouse with you." He appeared far different than he had when mired in depression years before, but he still maintained the same barriers that cut him off from help. In two sessions of lysergic acid diethylamide (LSD) therapy—an experimental approach to treatment at the time—his psychiatrist sought to break down these walls. Although the drug produced an "increase in his ability to relate to the therapist ... there did not seem to be any convincing evidence that he planned to change his life pattern," according to records of those sessions. Jim left the hospital with his poor prognosis unchanged. His psychiatrist wrote, "He has found that he is able to manipulate others through his generally antisocial behavior, which is impulsive and attention-seeking. He fits all the diagnostic criteria of the antisocial reaction."

Like Jim's, Doug's psychiatric evaluation and treatment (at age 29) reflected the theories and practices of the day, some of which have since been discarded by mainstream psychiatry. He was described as boyish-looking and reserved, cooperating well and displaying "no unusual mannerisms." The doctors focused on his sexual impulses and his intense fear of getting caught in some shameful act. They probed his early childhood experiences and were intrigued to find that his mother had bathed him until age 10, focusing "much attention on his penis." Psychoanalytic theory, with its emphasis on childhood sexuality, was prevalent at the time, and although it probably revealed little about Doug's antisocial personality, it may have shed light on his sexual confusion. He admitted taking every chance he could to spot his mother naked and felt that his window peeping stemmed from this early thrill. His doctors wove a psychoanalytic thread into their description of Doug's behavior, which, in their view, had developed to "satisfy some inner need .... He is unable to comprehend the reasons for his actions, but admits that voyeurism is exciting and dangerous and his sexual deviation is but one manifestation. He also shows a need for immediate gratification of his wishes [and] routine is intolerable. He lacks aim and foresight." They also noted his inability to withstand criticism, which was attributed to his excessive reaction and unexpressed hostility to a critical father.

Doug also received treatment with an experimental LSD-like drug called Ditran (piperidyl benzilate) that was thought to facilitate insight during therapy. Some psychiatrists, including the late Charles Shagass of the University of Iowa, also claimed that treatment with such hallucinogenic drugs could induce periods of remission in antisocials.[10] In Doug's case, the experiment seems to have added little to his therapy. He was diagnosed with "sociopathic personality, sexual deviation" and given a "most unfavorable" prognosis. Doug left the hospital after three months, mildly improved and less subject to "inner tension," according to his records.

Doug's diagnosis probably would be somewhat different today, at least in the way it was phrased. The *DSM-I*, the diagnostic manual used when he was evaluated in 1963, placed sexual deviation—in this case, window peeping—in a subcategory of sociopathic (later antisocial) personality. We now know that most people with sexual deviations are probably not antisocial, although Doug (and Paul in the last chapter) is an obvious exception. Today, Doug's voyeurism would likely supplement the main diagnosis of ASP. In light of his tendency toward self-mutilation, a diagnosis of *borderline personality disorder*—a condition characterized by emotional instability, impulsive behavior, and self-inflicted injuries, such as wrist cutting—might also be considered.

The experiences of Doug and Jim in the early to mid-1960s show how psychiatry has evolved. Today, Jim's clinical depression would likely be treated with antidepressant medication. Doug's therapy might focus less on what doctors thought his parents had done wrong and more on his own thought patterns and resulting behaviors.

WHAT HAPPENS TO ANTISOCIAL ADULTS?

Based on what happened to her study subjects, Robins concluded in *Deviant Children Grown Up* that ASP is a chronic, persistent disorder that seldom remits. Of the original 524 child guidance clinic patients in her study, 94 were identified as antisocial in adulthood, 82 of whom were interviewed in their 30s and 40s. Only 12% had remitted, showing no evidence of antisocial behavior. Another 27% had improved but were still getting into trouble, whereas fully 61% had not improved at all. In fact, some were considered worse.[11]

In my study, briefly described in Chapter 1, we were able to rate the outcome of 45 antisocial men (from an original sample of 71) who had been hospitalized years earlier and who were in their mid-50s at the time of our follow-up.[12] Using roughly the same ratings Robins used, we found that 27% had remitted and 31% had improved, but that the largest group—42%—showed no improvement. Four men were actually worse than they had been when originally hospitalized. Some of these men are described throughout this book, and, although their outcomes vary, most of their stories show that ASP has a lifelong impact even when those afflicted with it improve.

In Robins's study, the median age for improvement was 35 years, but she added a hopeful note that there was "no age beyond which improvement seemed impossible." Just because a subject had improved, however, did not mean that his disorder was no longer a problem, an observation that held true with my study subjects as well. Robins writes:

> The finding that more than one-third of the sociopathic group had given up much of the antisocial behavior ... does not mean that at present they are strikingly well-adjusted and agreeable persons. Many of them report interpersonal difficulties, irritability, hostility toward wives, neighbors, and organized religion.

They are in many cases no longer either a threat to the life and property of others nor a financial drain on society.[13]

Robins's conclusion that a sizable percentage of antisocials mellow with age is consistent with crime statistics showing that arrests peak among individuals in their late teens and decline as offenders grow older. Very few arrests occur in persons aged 60 or older, and those that do occur are more likely due to conduct offenses like public drunkenness rather than violent crime.[14]

The apparent burnout among antisocials has been enshrined in psychiatric literature despite little consensus on what it means and even if it truly occurs. The word *burnout* implies that antisocial behavior decreases to a point at which it is no longer a problem, like a light bulb dimming until its glow fades altogether. That said, although aging antisocials are less troublesome—at least to society as a whole—and are less likely to be arrested, few are model citizens. Sometimes the circle of others affected by their behavior merely tightens, involving just immediate family, or perhaps neighbors and co-workers. Although escaping arrest, they can cause trouble in different but no less destructive ways, lashing out in domestic violence or failing to provide adequate support for children. Even in old age, many of these men draw on public resources for survival. Those who age behind bars require greater care and sometimes special facilities. Those who live free may need extra help to compensate for a lack of financial resources and failing health exacerbated by years of irresponsible living. Even when its more striking symptoms taper off, ASP remains a lifelong disorder. Many of those who improve are unable to regain lost opportunities in education, employment, and domestic life and, for some, remission means continuing to live on society's margins. Like several of the men in this book, antisocials often spend their last years alone, sometimes troubled with regret for what they never knew they were missing until it was too late.

WHO IMPROVES?

When one asks an antisocial who has remitted, as my colleagues and I did, to explain his improvement, the answer can be surprising. Some cite increasing age or maturity, others marriage or the support of a loyal spouse. Still others attribute their change to fear of punishment or jail, or to increased responsibilities at home or at work. Religious conversions or other significant events that alter perspectives on life can also play a part. Mentors—whether spouses, employers, clergy, parents, or others—seem important in helping many people change their ways, although this influence is hard to measure.

Clearly, some antisocials improve, but the reasons are difficult to gauge, making it hard to predict which ones will improve or what will trigger the change. Robins relates a number of characteristics to improvement, beginning with age. She found that antisocials older than 40 were more likely to have improved than their younger counterparts, suggesting that remission is a matter of time for some. In my own outcomes research, age and time also emerged as significant factors tied to improvement. The oldest men I contacted for follow-up interviews were the most likely to show improvement, as were those for whom the most years had elapsed since their hospitalizations, particularly if they had stopped drinking.[15]

Robins found that marriage and incarceration both have an effect on ASP. Few of the single antisocials she studied had improved compared to more than half of the married ones. Spouses, partners, and others close to the antisocial can play an important role in urging therapy, and improvement often comes when one has a source of personal support and motivation. Antisocials who remitted had stronger family ties, were more involved in their communities, and were more likely to live with their wives. These findings are largely consistent with the Gluecks' findings that linked job stability and marital attachment with improvement.[16] Looking at incarceration, Robins found that men jailed for less than a year had a higher rate of remission than both those who had never been to jail and those who spent longer periods behind bars, indicating that brief incarceration acts as a deterrent for some.

Of course, each of these situations—from brief incarceration to relative success with marriage and family life—could easily be the *result* of improvement rather than its cause. One might expect that antisocials who stay happily married, or who have not faced lengthy periods of incarceration, have milder cases of ASP to begin with or are otherwise predisposed to getting better. There is some evidence for this, at least with regard to marriage. In a study of male twins followed from age 17 to 29, the researchers discovered that men with *less* severe forms of antisocial behavior were more likely to marry than their more antisocial brothers. Possibly, severe antisocial symptoms hinder marriage because they interfere with forming intimate relationships.[17]

Some researchers have looked for fundamental risk factors that may limit an antisocial's chances for improvement. In my own work, the most important variable has been the severity of ASP in early adulthood. Just as children with the earliest and most serious behavior problems are most likely to develop ASP, young adults with the most varied and severe symptoms remain in the grip of their disorder the longest. Again, it would seem that some cases are simply worse than others or that some antisocials establish an early pattern that is more difficult to shake loose.

ANTISOCIAL PERSONALITY DISORDER AND OTHER PSYCHIATRIC DISORDERS

Contrary to early writers like Cleckley, who believed that few of his psychopaths developed problems like depression or an anxiety disorder, research shows that ASP is strongly linked with other mental illnesses.[18] Depression and anxiety are part of the problem, but antisocials also are at high risk for alcoholism and drug dependency, attention-deficit/hyperactivity disorder (ADHD), sexual deviancy, pathological gambling, and other conditions. Therefore, a diagnosis of ASP raises the possibility of additional mental health problems, whether as aspects of a patient's past or as future risks.

Among the clearest of these links is the one between ASP and the *abuse of alcohol or other drugs*.[19] Nearly 84% of antisocials surveyed in the Epidemiologic Catchment Area (ECA) study had some form of alcohol or drug abuse during their lifetime. Uncontrolled substance use exacerbates other symptoms associated with ASP, often bringing out the worst in an individual's personality. The violent antisocial is more apt to lash out; the philanderer loses any remaining inhibition. For this reason, encouraging the antisocial to deal with his alcohol or drug use is an important first step in any treatment program.

Substance abuse also complicates the diagnosis of ASP. Some researchers maintain that ASP cannot be accurately diagnosed in alcoholics or drug addicts, as it is hard to tell where intoxication and addiction end and personality disorder begins. I disagree, and believe that, with the true antisocial, telltale signs of ASP will be found in the patient's history and include evidence of childhood conduct disorder and problems in adult life that continue even through periods of sobriety.[20]

Antisocials may also be at increased risk for other addictive or compulsive behaviors that don't involve drugs or alcohol, notably *pathological gambling*.[21] Although gambling has shed much of its shady image, it remains tied to antisocial behavior. Both alcoholism and ASP are overrepresented among habitual gamblers, most of whom are men. The accessibility of lotteries, casinos, and other forms of betting has made compulsive gambling more pervasive, and awareness of the problem has accompanied the growth in legalized gambling. Promises of instant gratification and excitement, without regard for consequences, may draw antisocials into gambling because their personalities are already fine-tuned to such appeals. Coupled with his near complete irresponsibility and lack of regard for the needs of his family members, the antisocial can easily be drawn into the web of pathological gambling and its promise of easy riches, thus bringing financial disaster to all.

Mood disorders are another significant risk for one-third to one-half of antisocials. Some, like Jim, develop *major depressive disorder,* also known as *clinical depression.* The mood disorders *dysthymia* (chronic low-level depression) and *bipolar disorder* (with its characteristic extreme highs and lows) and anxiety states like *panic disorder, social phobia, posttraumatic stress disorder,* and *obsessive-compulsive disorder (OCD)* are also quite common. Whether due to a biological predisposition or an understandable response to their all too often miserable lives, severe depression drives many people with ASP to attempt suicide. About 5% eventually succeed—compared to 1% of the general population. Death by suicide—an outcome Cleckley thought rare—turns out to be relatively common.[22]

Many antisocials have a history of childhood ADHD, a condition with effects that can linger into adulthood.[23] Childhood ADHD is characterized by impulsiveness, hyperactivity, and inability to sustain attention, and its symptoms overlap with those of conduct disorder. The two conditions are often concurrent, although the presence of one may mask the other. Rachel Gittelman and her colleagues studied 101 boys and young men with ADHD at the New York State Psychiatric Institute 10 years after their initial childhood evaluations and found a link between ADHD and ASP. At follow-up, 27% of the subjects had either conduct disorder or ASP, depending on their ages. Nineteen percent—most of them in the conduct disorder/ASP category—also abused drugs or alcohol. The researchers concluded that many of the boys with ADHD who had also exhibited delinquent behavior went on to develop ASP. When ADHD remains a problem in adult life, psychostimulant medications like methylphenidate (Ritalin) may paradoxically have a calming effect and allay symptoms, as they do in children with ADHD.

A particularly interesting phenomenon—notable for its relationship to gender—is the link between ASP and *somatization disorder*.[24] A bizarre illness once called *hysteria*, somatization disorder usually develops during early adulthood and is characterized by multiple physical complaints—headaches, numbness, breathing problems, generalized aches and pains—that lack a medical explanation. The disorder is particularly common in antisocial women, and some theorize that it may be a female counterpart to the largely male ASP. A case can be made for a genetic link between the two disorders, as somatization disorder is unusually common among female relatives of male criminals. It is possible that a common genetic quirk mediated by biological and cultural differences leads to different psychiatric disorders in men and women. Some psychiatrists also hypothesize that the symptoms of somatization disorder limit the behaviors associated with ASP, as they render a woman too "sick" to act out.

Other unusual psychiatric disorders may appear in conjunction with ASP. *Factitious disorders* are a curious group of conditions in which individuals feign or simulate physical or mental illness for no apparent reason other than to assume a sick role. One patient may simply rub a thermometer to give the impression of fever. Another may go to extreme lengths, like an inpatient I once treated who injected feces into his knee joint to induce an infection. Factitious disorders can be difficult to diagnose and may force physicians to match wits with clever patients to catch them in the act of faking symptoms.

Malingering, on the other hand, is the term used when people exaggerate or simulate illness for obvious reasons, perhaps trying to avoid work or obtain medications. One notorious malingerer was Kenneth Bianchi, also known as the "Hillside Strangler."[25]

He attempted to escape execution for the rape and murder of 10 women by feigning multiple personality disorder but was ultimately found out. It comes as no surprise that many malingerers are antisocial. They enjoy duping doctors and nurses and are skillful deceivers who may require close observation if they are to be caught. In their book *Patient or Pretender*, psychiatrists Marc Feldman and Charles Ford tell of a woman who faked ovarian cancer. She moved in with her boyfriend and proceeded to fleece him of his savings, drink excessively, and complain of pain and exhaustion. After a heated argument one night, she told him about her "cancer." Although feeling guilty at first for having doubted her complaints, he soon began to suspect her vague descriptions of "treatment" and lack of physical changes, finally discovering her history of feigned illnesses. She threatened his life when confronted. The authors concluded that the woman had ASP and that her "web of lies goes beyond a reckless disregard for the truth.... The woman showed no remorse."[26]

A topic that deserves special consideration with regard to ASP is sexual deviance, or *paraphilia*. The term applies to any preference for inappropriate or dangerous patterns of sexual arousal, and ranges from relatively harmless but annoying behaviors like exhibitionism or voyeurism to severe and destructive conditions like pedophilia. Abnormal sexual desires and behaviors have long been associated with ASP, but we now know that most antisocials are not sexually deviant, although paraphilias are more common among them than in the general population.[27] It is also important to note that what psychiatry and society regard as harmful sexual activity has been known to change with time and context. Homosexuality, for instance, was once considered a psychiatric disturbance, but sexual orientation is now understood to be an innate human characteristic that should otherwise be of little interest to mental health professionals unless it leads to distress.[28] When men like Doug and James were evaluated in the early 1960s, however, the same sex incidents in their past likely were used to bolster their psychiatrists' findings.

Many sexual characteristics and tastes are considered benign by most psychiatrists so long as they don't complicate life for the individuals who possess them. Of course, the problem with some paraphilias is the possibility that they will lead to harming other people. The issue of pedophilia and sexual predators who do serious physical and emotional damage to children is perhaps the best example of public and professional concern over sexual deviance. The pedophile not only offends our protective instincts toward children, but also acts out of a desire that is commonly regarded as untreatable, making him a perpetual threat. But most active pedophiles are not antisocial; sex is often the main area of life where their deviancy emerges, and, apart from that, they may present a veneer of normalcy.

Violent sex offenders have inspired recent efforts to curtail their crimes and impose harsher punishments, including longer prison terms for first-time convictions and the controversial method of "chemical castration," in which convicted criminals are administered drugs that diminish sex drive. New Jersey legislators passed "Megan's Law"—a measure requiring that communities be notified when a sex offender settles in their midst—after Jesse Timmendequas raped and killed young Megan Kanka.[29] The law has been duplicated in many other states, as have laws permitting the confinement of dangerous sex offenders beyond the length of their prison terms, often in mental hospitals. The State of Washington passed such a law after Earl Shriner kidnapped a seven-year-old boy, raped and stabbed him, and cut off his penis. Shriner had served time for child molestation before but was released at the end of his sentence, even though authorities knew he was still dangerous.[30]

Most psychiatrists, including myself, oppose the indefinite commitment of sex offenders to mental hospitals, despite a 1997 Supreme Court decision that ruled these laws constitutional.[31] At issue was a Kansas law permitting some criminals to be forcibly hospitalized after serving their prison terms if their behavior stemmed from a "mental abnormality or personality disorder" that made them likely to engage in further crimes. Those who commit sex crimes fit no particular psychiatric profile or treatment plan, and although various therapies for sex offenders have been developed, there is little consensus regarding their effectiveness and ability to maintain public safety. Offenders hospitalized under these laws could end up institutionalized for life, burdening already underfunded public mental hospitals. Furthermore, hospitals do not provide the security found in prisons, and truly dangerous criminals should remain under the watch of corrections officers, not doctors.

The rape of adults is another sexual crime that rouses concern, although the relationship between rape and paraphilia—and between rape and ASP—remains problematic. Many regard rape as a crime of violence, despite its undeniable sexual component. Some men are serial rapists, driven by violent sexual urges, but other rapes are isolated acts driven by alcohol, drugs, opportunity, and other factors. Certainly, rape and other sex crimes are important aspects of the criminal history for some men with ASP, and it may be the case that antisocial men, with their tendency to defy social regulation, are more likely to commit rape than are others.

FOLLOW-UPS

In late 1988, Cathy Butler managed to find Jim through the State Division of Motor Vehicles. Since he had no phone, she contacted him by certified mail to request that he take part in our study. An unusual correspondence followed as Jim kept seeking more information about the study in letters that revealed his strange blend of interest and irritation. "I am not big on B.S., so get your stuff together," he wrote. "I'm too old to play games." He seemed to enjoy toying with us, questioning the validity of our work, accusing us of ignorance, and insisting that a personal interview would be possible only if we went to him. As an alternative, he suggested that we provide him a free week of hospitalization to facilitate "more in-depth interviews." Cathy finally arranged a meeting, and he sent a map of his town along with pamphlets on antique glassware that he had self-published 20 years before. "I will be waiting," he wrote.

More than a year earlier, Sue Bell, my other researcher, had found Doug living in a small Iowa town. Her timing was perfect. Doug quickly agreed to an interview when she called, commenting that his wife was away at a wedding in New Mexico. She knew little of his past, he said, and he wanted to keep it that way. Had she been home, he would have declined the telephone interview. Classical music played in the background as Doug fielded Sue's questions. Had he been arrested since his hospitalization 24 years earlier? Ten to 12 times, he reported, with at least four felony convictions, the last a 1973 breaking-and-entering charge that carried a four-year prison term. Had he been hospitalized again? Three times for depression and once for a 10-month alcohol treatment program, he said, adding that his last hospitalization was in 1971. Did he still window peep? "Heavens no," Doug insisted, "that stopped years ago." Sue recorded his answer, although she remained suspicious. A 1974 competency evaluation done in connection with a burglary charge stated that Doug was sexually attracted to his mother, "considers himself bisexual, and has a history of window-peeping, exhibitionism, and pedophilia towards the children of his third wife. It was for this reason he was committed as a sexual psychopath … for seven months." Sue doubted that his sex offenses had completely ended, even after nearly 15 years.

A telephone interview was not an option for Cathy's follow-up with Jim, and although she preferred to meet with subjects in person, the interviews sometimes took her to bleak and even frightening surroundings. Something about Jim had roused her defenses, but she was relieved to find his town a charming strip of antique shops and specialty stores. Jim lived above one such shop, run by an older woman who peered from the window as Cathy stepped from her car and pulled her coat tight against the December air. She found an entrance and stairs leading to the upper floors and waited for someone to answer her knock at Jim's apartment door. The man who appeared identified himself as Jim's half-stepbrother and said Jim must have forgotten the interview. He offered to find him while Cathy waited in the shop below. Downstairs, the proprietor apologized for the suspicious glance she had shot Cathy before, explaining that the emblem on Cathy's university car had prompted her concern. "I just knew social services would be here before long," she said, gesturing to the ceiling and the apartments above. Cathy asked what she meant, and the woman explained that her tenant, Jim, was a chronic alcoholic well known by bartenders and police alike. He was friendly enough, she said, but spent his days panhandling and often got into trouble.

Jim arrived more than an hour later, a stooped man with thinning hair who appeared much older than his 56 years. He invited Cathy upstairs to his smelly rooms. Plaster flaked from the ceiling, and a battered radiator sighed a constant hiss of steam. Tattered newspapers, drained liquor bottles, and greasy heaps of clothing were strewn over the floor. A bottle labeled "marital stimulant pills" sat on a table next to the stained sofa, and Cathy wondered if it had been placed there deliberately. She and Jim sat facing each other across a small dining table. He urged her to make herself comfortable, but his crooked smile kept her nervous. "You'd better hurry up," he said. "I have important things to do."

He had received an English degree at the University of Nebraska and had spent 28 years selling antiques on the street, Jim reported with obvious pride. Cathy remembered what the woman downstairs had said about his panhandling and surmised that Jim's business must be quite slow, if it existed at all. He told her he lived with help from Food Stamps and looked forward to receiving veterans' benefits. On a friend's advice, he was seeing a psychiatrist in an effort to demonstrate emotional problems that might qualify him for additional aid, but when Cathy asked him to describe his problems, he merely smiled and waited until she moved on to the next question. Had he ever been arrested, she asked? Not for 10 years, Jim maintained, and before that only three times, an account that bore only scant resemblance to his record of selling drugs, carrying a concealed weapon, simple assault, criminal trespass, and other crimes listed on his rap sheet. By this time, Cathy had noticed the fading light outside and suggested that they continue the interview at a later date. They arranged a February meeting, and Jim saw her out. She descended the stairs and hurried to her car, glad to be away from Jim and his filthy, dimly lit apartment.

Jim's situation at follow-up was a far cry from Doug's, although problems had continued for both men. The latter, Sue learned, worked part-time for a local newspaper and performed odd jobs, including painting and landscape work. Nevertheless, Doug and his wife could barely scrape by and received state aid in the winter to pay for their heat. He said they had once taken Food Stamps as well, but the necessary paperwork and the embarrassment of using the coupons at local stores had prompted them to stop. He recalled that his best job had been on the kill line at a local meat-packing plant that had since closed. After that, he had worked briefly as a school janitor. His current wife was his fifth, and he confessed he had sometimes been cruel to the women he lived with, usually after drinking. He and his wife had fought for a while, but things had calmed down in the 11 years since their wedding, in part, he said, because he had learned to handle his temper. He had fathered one son in his first marriage, but had lost contact with him and had never helped with child support. He said nothing about the second, illegitimate child that we knew had resulted from an extramarital affair.

When asked to describe his sexual identity, Doug replied that he was definitely bisexual, and that the only love he had ever felt was for another man during his stay at the Patuxent Institute. Infrequent homosexual contacts had followed, always kept secret from his wives. Doug surprised Sue with the astonishing remark that his life might have been better had he been born a woman. He would have been more comfortable, he maintained, although he suspected that he might have taken up prostitution. His sex drive was still strong, he said, describing it as a "sort of tension." His regular labor kept him physically healthy, although his past injuries included knife and gunshot wounds, both of which he attributed to fights. The shooting, we learned, actually occurred when he was running from police after a burglary, an incident he claimed to have forgotten but noted in the 1974 competency evaluation mentioned earlier. Doug's scarce social outlets included membership in a local chess club, although he and his wife largely kept to themselves in their rented home.

Sue asked whether he had settled down, and he replied that, yes, his life had changed. "I'm far too old to live that way anymore," he said with a tinge of nostalgia. "I'm not as quick as I used to be." Was he still reckless? Sometimes, he admitted, refusing to elaborate. Giving up alcohol, which he had finally managed to do on his own, had brought the most significant changes, he said. He had come to the point where he wanted control of his life, and he ended the interview with an observation that he had wasted many of his years and abilities. With his intelligence, he said, he could have accomplished so much more.

Unlike Doug, Jim was unwilling—perhaps unable—to look back on his life with even a hint of insight. When Cathy returned for their second interview, he was waiting for her outside the building, despite the freezing cold. He led her up the stairs to the apartment, visibly steadying himself against the banister and giggling as she unpacked her interview materials. She saw that he was smoking and began with an easy question: Have you ever smoked cigarettes daily for a month or more? "No," he said, his giggles erupting into full-blown laughter that he quelled with a sip of something that looked like water. "But you're smoking now," she pointed out. He claimed that he smoked only when on drinking binges, and Cathy asked if he was currently bingeing. "I've been drinking for 15 days straight and I'm not about to stop," he declared, and produced a bottle of vodka from under the table. "Want some?" he asked, waving the bottle in Cathy's direction before putting it to his lips and taking a huge swig. She declined his offer.

Although she had barely begun, Cathy told Jim she was ending the interview and had to be on her way. She shuffled her papers together and avoided his eyes. "I know why you came here," he said. "You want me as bad as I want you." By now, Cathy was on her feet and headed for the door. Jim followed and managed to back her into a corner, then took the cigarette from his mouth and poked its ember at her face. She screamed and brought her knee up hard against his groin, sending him sprawling across the carpet and gasping for air. On her way down the staircase, she could hear him kicking his legs against the floor and laughing with drunken glee.

Jim had clearly grown worse with time, whereas Doug was somewhat improved. Although he still had more than his share of problems—a largely loveless marriage, a low income, an unstable work history, and a general dissatisfaction with life—he claimed to have given up crime and drinking. Jim, however, was hopelessly reliant on alcohol. There was no indication that his youthful pleas for help, no matter how vague and inconsistent, were being voiced any longer, and the isolation he had tried to overcome as a child and young adult was now his way of life. Doug at least was able to function after decades of dealing with ASP and had even begun to understand what he had lost in his tumultuous years of lies, crime, and self-destructiveness. However, his regrets revolved around himself, and he expressed no remorse for abusing his wives, abandoning his children, and otherwise hurting those around him. Neither Doug nor Jim had remitted—not even coming close—but their lives had veered in different directions, Doug's edging up, Jim's down. Their lives show how the course of ASP can vary from case to case and why predicting the natural history of the disorder is not an exact science.

Jim's case in particular shows why research into ASP can be so challenging. Cathy's brush with terror in his run-down apartment caused us to rethink the wisdom of sending a single interviewer to meet with potentially dangerous subjects. Her presence of mind averted tragedy that day, but working with antisocials always carries an element of risk. Their unpredictability and capacity for violence make antisocials difficult to study and may help explain why few researchers choose to focus on this disorder.

Chapter 6

Seeds of Despair

The Causes of
Antisocial Personality Disorder

NATURE AND NURTURE

Bad parenting, defective genes, childhood trauma, poverty—these are but a few of the proposed causal factors in antisocial personality disorder (ASP), a list as varied as the selection of experts who stand behind their favorite explanations for the disorder. Just as the diverse manifestations of ASP may divert attention from the underlying disorder, focusing on a single cause risks overlooking the possibility that ASP results from combinations of factors. The sociologist blames the poor living conditions found in deteriorating inner cities or rural backwaters. The psychologist regards ASP as a learned behavior that impressionable children pick up from bad parents. The psychiatrist views the disorder as being hereditary and biologically driven. The psychoanalyst sees inconsistent parenting in early childhood as having lifelong effects. This list is something of a caricature, but it underlines the fact that ASP probably has multiple causes. Although we lack the knowledge to name definitive causes of the disorder, we know enough to suggest various factors that may contribute to its development.

Interesting and certainly important, the question of causation must be kept in perspective. Most mental illnesses cannot be attributed to any particular cause. We know of no virus, for instance, that causes schizophrenia, no genetic mutation that results in depression. At present, psychiatry is unable to explain fully the origins of *any* mental illness (save for minor exceptions, such as stroke-related dementia). These complex and variable illnesses are difficult to trace back to their sources, but uncertain cause does not prevent us from confronting them. Encountering a patient who fits the criteria for ASP, I can never say with certainty where his problems come from, but I can still describe possible outcomes and offer treatment options. We may never fully understand the causes of ASP, but what we do find may lead to advances in treatment or prevention.

Most of the debate about the causes of mental illness—as well as of other human conditions—tends to swirl around the relative influence of nature versus nurture, or heredity versus environment. In this context, *nature* is generally construed as genetics and biology, whereas *nurture* refers to home and social environment plus early life experiences. Those favoring genetic theories for ASP point to families in which patterns of misbehavior are repeated from generation to generation, suggesting a hereditary influence rooted in biology. Those favoring nurture see in the same families cycles of deprivation and abuse that lead to similar behavior in parents and children. In reality, the nature–nurture debate over ASP and other conditions is largely spurious. Individuals who could be genetically predisposed to ASP may express their tendencies in learned behaviors like neglect or physical abuse. A family history of these behaviors could reflect hereditary as well as environmental influences. In the end, the most satisfying theories of causation tread a middle ground between nature and nurture, drawing elements from both.

The heredity–environment debate is hardly new, especially in psychiatry, but revolutionary progress in genetics today weighs one side of the equation more heavily than ever before. Genes tied to traits like novelty-seeking, aggression, and sexual orientation have been proposed, sometimes raising furious controversy. Even characteristics with obvious genetic links are often more complex than many tend to think. Genetics may set the potential, but environmental factors, such as diet and family upbringing, may determine whether that potential is ultimately reached. Few question, for example, that height is influenced by genes, but environmental influences also play a clear role. Japanese Americans are taller than their Japanese parents, probably because of differences in diet, not genes.[1] Weight provides another example of gene–environment interaction. An individual who inherits a gene related to obesity will not become fat without the necessary caloric intake. Similarly, I think it is best to view ASP as the result of an underlying genetic predisposition that is shaped and molded by environmental and social forces.

ORIGINS

In early 1990, Ruben Deases, age 18, was sentenced to life in prison for the gruesome murder and mutilation of a young woman in Iowa. His 22-year-old brother, Edward, awaited trial for the same crime, witnessed by a third, younger brother who exchanged his testimony for immunity. Jurors heard accounts of how the woman was murdered and how one of the killers allegedly had sex with her corpse. The body was eventually beheaded and quickly discarded, and the murderers reportedly made up rap songs about the victim after the crime. She had been the girlfriend of yet another Deases brother, who was jailed for cocaine trafficking at the time. Two additional brothers had had brushes with the law and, while growing up, four of the six Deases boys had spent time at Boys' Town, the famous home for troubled youth near Omaha, Nebraska. Their offenses ranged from auto theft to drug crimes.

The case received wide attention in the Iowa media, and the *Des Moines Register* ran an in-depth piece tracing patterns of violence through the Deases family.[2] A sister of the boys recounted a terrifying childhood with an alcoholic father, claiming that he regularly beat his sons and ran up gambling debts that brought danger and despair to their home. She explained how the elder Deases also beat his wife, once throwing her in a ditch and pummeling her when she was eight months pregnant. Questioned about such abuse, the father, Alfred Deases, admitted hitting his children for discipline and explained that his own father had raised him in the same manner. He described watching his father strangle an infant who would not stop crying. She died the next day. Alfred Deases added that one of his brothers had been crippled by childhood abuse and that a sister received permanent burn scars when her hands were held over a hot surface.

In courtrooms and newspapers, experts commenting on the Deases case debated the influence of such abuse on criminal behavior, some suggesting that it ultimately led to the murder. The view that childhood beatings almost inevitably lead to additional violence later in life—a widely held perception—was frequently counterbalanced by fear or outrage that such an explanation might be used to excuse the most grievous criminal behavior. Absent were discussions of why such violence occurs across generations of families. I do not know whether any of the Deases men have been or could be diagnosed with ASP, but their story shows how antisocial symptoms often travel in families. Violence and other problems associated with ASP often are shared by parents and children, from excessive drinking to troubles with school or work.

Like the Deases boys, men with ASP often have family histories that reveal clues to hereditary and environmental factors that can influence behavior. Some, like Jim in the last chapter, have family members whose behavior sounds suspiciously antisocial. Although he never knew his father, Jim grew up thinking of the man as a wanderer who abandoned his boys, charting a path that Jim would eventually follow. Others, like Doug, have clear-cut family histories of ASP or other disorders. In an early evaluation, a psychiatrist noted that Doug's mother was a hypochondriac who once had been hospitalized for "simple adult maladjustment." Psychiatric records described her as impulsive and subject to uncontrollable emotional outbursts. Doug's father was an alcoholic who had been sent to reform school as a youth, and his two younger brothers were both intellectually challenged, an observation that may or may not bear any relation to Doug's behavior problems. Whatever the link, both antisocial behavior and antisocial personality often run in families, and it is here that the search for causes usually begins.

THE APPLE FALLS NEAR THE TREE

The idea that bad behavior might somehow be "in the genes" has long been a topic for science and the popular imagination. The 1956 film *The Bad Seed*, based on the novel by William March, depicts a malicious young girl who kills a classmate at a school picnic to obtain a medal he won. The murder is not her first, nor is it unprecedented in her family, as the film reveals that the girl's father—a man she had never met—was also a killer. Raised by a kind, caring mother, the girl could not have learned her murderous ways at home. She must therefore be the product of a "bad seed," an inevitable tendency toward violence inherited from an absent father.

Stories like this feed a common fear about mental illness—the concern that it can be passed genetically from parent to child. The fear is potentially justified for many serious psychiatric disorders (and many physical ailments as well). Genetics unquestionably plays a role in schizophrenia, bipolar disorder, alcoholism, anxiety disorders, and several other mental health conditions. But the simple fact that a disorder like ASP or a characteristic like criminal behavior runs in families does not prove genetic causation. I have a close friend who is a psychiatrist, as were his father and his father's sister, but surely my friend's career choice was not genetically determined. He may have inherited attributes that were helpful in his education and work, such as a tendency to be achievement-oriented, but these traits could just as easily been taught or otherwise fostered by his family.

To establish evidence for a link between genes and a particular psychiatric disorder, researchers take several routes of investigation, including studies of families, twins, and adoptees. Family studies typically involve evaluation of first-degree relatives—parents, siblings, and children—of people who display the disorder in question and who share 50% of their genes. Researchers ascertain whether the disorder is more common among first-degree relatives of people in whom it has been diagnosed than among relatives of a healthy control group. If rates of the disorder are higher among relatives of those with the illness, the results suggest that the disorder runs in families and is possibly genetic. Family studies of ASP have generally shown that nearly 20%—one in five—of antisocials' first-degree relatives are themselves antisocial and that between one-quarter and one-third are alcoholic.[3] Depression, drug abuse, somatization disorder, attention-deficit/hyperactivity disorder (ADHD), and learning disabilities also run in these families. Male relatives of antisocials are more likely to have ASP, alcoholism or drug dependency, ADHD, and learning disabilities, whereas female relatives more commonly suffer from depression or somatization disorder, a condition characterized by multiple, unexplained medical complaints. Taken together, family studies of ASP indicate that children with an antisocial parent have about a 16% chance of developing the disorder.

Although these studies suggest that ASP runs in families, they fail to answer questions about the influence of genetics. Environmental factors alone could increase the chances that a child will follow in his antisocial parent's footsteps, perhaps learning behaviors or acting out in response to neglect and abuse. To disentangle the effects of heredity and environment, researchers turn to studies of twins and adopted children. Twin studies usually begin with pairs of identical and nonidentical (fraternal) siblings in which one of the twins is known to have a particular mental illness. The other twin is then assessed to determine whether he or she also has the disorder. If a disorder is more commonly shared by identical twins than by nonidentical twins, it is thought to have a stronger genetic basis since identical twins carry the same genetic material. In theory, nonidentical twins share only 50% of their genes, so a disorder that is completely genetic would be found in both twins roughly 50% of the time, whereas its concordance rate in identical twins would be close to 100%. So far, the combined results of twin studies of ASP and criminal behavior reveal concordance rates of 67% in identical twins and 31% in non-identical twins, strongly supporting genetic theories of causation.[4] But these findings also leave room for environmental factors, because the concordance rate remains significantly below 100% for identical twins.

Adoption studies take the search for genetic links in a different direction. They look at the biological children of parents with a particular mental illness who were adopted and reared by presumably normal parents. By studying adoptees, researchers can discount the effects of learned behavior and role modeling that might occur if the children were raised by their mentally ill biological parents. If children adopted from parents with mental illness develop the same disorder more frequently than a control group of adopted children born to normal parents, a degree of genetic causation has been shown. In general, children of criminal or antisocial parents are more likely than other children to exhibit criminal or antisocial behavior as adults, even when early adoption removes them from the negative influence of their biological parents. Raymond Crowe, a psychiatrist and colleague of mine at the University of Iowa, studied a group of 52 adoptees born to 41 female criminals, managing to find 46 of the adoptees after an extensive search.[5] Six of them—or 13%—were diagnosed as antisocial, compared to only 2% of control adoptees. The children of female criminals also tended to have more serious arrest records that included more offenses, convictions, and incarcerations than the control group.

Adoption studies usually begin with parents who have a particular disorder, but a twist on the strategy involves tracking down the biological and adoptive relatives of mentally ill adoptees. Conducted in the 1960s and 1970s, the Danish Adoption Study is perhaps the largest and most complex example of this method.[6] Since rules of confidentiality complicate such studies in the United States, investigators Seymour Kety, David Rosenthal, and Paul Wender turned to Denmark, a small country with relatively complete and accessible records. Among their wide-ranging goals was a study of ASP and genetics. After identifying antisocials who had been adopted as children, the research team investigated both biological and adoptive relatives to compare rates of the disorder. They found ASP to be much more common among those who were related to antisocial adoptees by blood, again suggesting a genetic predisposition to antisocial behavior and personality.

The late Remi Cadoret, another psychiatrist from the University of Iowa, devoted his career to studying adoptees and the effects of growing up in adoptive homes. In his adoption studies of ASP, Cadoret makes a compelling case that environment and genetics are intertwined. Studying 241 adoptees, 30 of them antisocial, he and his colleagues found that the antisocials were more likely to have antisocial biological relatives. But they also determined that a chaotic family life in the adoptive home—having adoptive relatives with ASP, adoptive parents who divorce, or low socioeconomic status—substantially boosted the risk of developing ASP. In another study of 197 adoptees, Cadoret found that these factors led to aggression and conduct disorder only in adoptees whose biological parents had ASP, whereas others at low genetic risk for the disorder were virtually unaffected by stress in the adoptive home.[7]

All of these studies suggest that—at least to some extent—ASP is genetically transmitted.[8] But exactly what is inherited? Is there an "ASP gene," and, if so, what does it cause to go wrong in those who develop the disorder? Similar questions are being asked about every major psychiatric disorder and countless physical ones. Molecular genetics is the science that seeks to identify the gene or genes that might produce an illness. In the case of Huntington's disease, studies of large Venezuelan families with unusually high rates of the disorder narrowed the search for its genetic origin to a specific region on the short arm of chromosome 4. Such discoveries are becoming increasingly common, but they may be a long time coming for disorders like ASP. For one thing, more than one gene may play a role in ASP, and different genes may be responsible for different aspects of the disorder. Complicating the search are disagreements about which antisocials to study. Do we look at hard-core criminals or mild antisocials? Those with depression or without? Psychopaths or nonpsychopaths? Finding study subjects is another challenge, because this type of research generally requires large families filled with antisocials, or the availability of hundreds—if not thousands—of antisocial subjects and their DNA. Either strategy faces significant challenges, not the least of which is that funding is difficult to come by. These large "multiplex" families would likely be uncooperative, and there is no guarantee that large numbers of antisocials would cooperate with a study to extract their genetic material either.

If science ever manages to locate such a gene, the search will not end there. The next step will be to determine what the gene products are and how they function at the cellular level to create a vulnerability to ASP.

SEROTONIN AND OTHER NEUROTRANSMITTERS

One area of intense interest to scientists probing the biological roots of antisocial behavior is serotonin and other neurotransmitters. Neurotransmitters are molecules that ferry messages from one nerve cell to a corresponding receptor on another cell, thus providing the chemical basis for every thought, emotion, and memory we experience. Among the 50 or so neurotransmitters that have been identified, serotonin is thought to play a special role in mediating violent and aggressive behavior. As such, it has prompted theories that antisocial behavior and personality may stem from a genetic disorder of serotonin function. This is not to say that serotonin is the only brain chemical involved in aggression—and certainly not the only player in ASP—for the brain's workings are much more complex than that. Serotonin could be a common endpoint of various pathways that are influenced by other neurotransmitters, such as dopamine and norepinephrine. It also has an important role in other behavioral and mood disorders, including depression, panic disorder, bulimia, and obsessive-compulsive disorder (OCD). Nonetheless, the "serotonin hypothesis" may help explain how a genetically encoded predisposition for antisocial behavior might intersect with the environment.

The initial breakthrough implicating serotonin in antisocial behavior came in 1976. In a brief report, Swedish psychiatrist Marie Åsberg and her colleagues described a group of impulsive suicide attempters whose cerebrospinal fluid (CSF)—which bathes the spinal cord and cushions the brain—had unusually low levels of 5-hydroxyindoleacetic acid (5-HIAA), the primary metabolite, or breakdown product, of serotonin.[9] In the years since their report, evidence linking serotonin to impulsive and violent behaviors of all types has mounted. At the National Institute of Mental Health, researchers found low levels of 5-HIAA in the CSF of 26 aggressive men, and Finnish scientists discovered similarly low levels in men who killed with unusual cruelty and/or committed arson.[10] Offenders whose crimes are premeditated appear to have normal levels of this brain metabolite, suggesting that abnormally low serotonin may facilitate rash or violent antisocial behavior rather than crime itself.

Although it may seem a stretch to link this finding—which has become one of the best replicated in biological psychiatry—to ASP itself, many, if not most, of the subjects in these studies were antisocial, and the target symptoms of impulsivity and violence are major aspects of the disorder. Additional evidence tying serotonin to aggression has accumulated. If tryptophan hydroxylase—an enzyme that directs the body's production of serotonin—in the blood is depleted, even normal men become more aggressive. Studies in mice show that they not only turn more aggressive when serotonin is depleted, but they also become more docile when the serotonin system is revved up. Finally, treatment studies have shown that violent outbursts or aggression may be modulated by drugs that boost serotonin levels. From these findings, I think it is reasonable to conclude that disturbed serotonin function plays a critical role in mediating antisocial behavior.[11]

Researchers still have a poor understanding of precisely how serotonin regulates impulses and aggression. In his book *Listening to Prozac*, psychiatrist Peter Kramer describes serotonin as having a policing role. Citing an unnamed researcher, Kramer writes, "If you don't have enough police, all sorts of things can happen. You may have riots. The absence of police does not cause riots. But if you do have a riot and you don't have the police, there is nothing to stop the riot from happening."[12] From an evolutionary perspective, the serotonin system likely developed early, creating a precarious balance essential to human survival. Too little and primal aggression would go unchecked. Too much and people would become overly passive, unable to manage life in the harsh world where early humans had to struggle for survival. People with inadequate serotonin levels may lack a necessary chemical resource for keeping impulsive and violent behavior in check, but the connection between serotonin and other psychiatric disorders implies that it is only part of the ASP story.

Monoamine oxidase (MAO), a major enzyme that breaks down serotonin, is another important aspect of the story. Considerable evidence has accumulated tying low MAO activity to aggressive behavior and criminality, both symptoms of ASP. Yet the precise role of MAO activity is unclear, because one might think that lower rates of serotonin breakdown would lead to higher levels of the neurotransmitter, which, as I have pointed out, is linked with *less* aggression. Regardless, MAO has become an even more interesting part of the

ASP story because a low activity variant of the gene that influences one type of monoamine—the MAOA genotype—has been found in antisocial persons who had been severely abused as children. In contrast, children who had a high-activity variant of the gene rarely became antisocial. Behavioral scientist Avshalom Caspi and colleagues had reported this in the prestigious journal *Science* in 2002. It set off a firestorm of interest because it represented the first time that not only was a specific gene tied to antisocial behavior, but the study made clear that *expression* of the bad behavior was linked to childhood abuse, clearly a nongenetic factor. Since that initial report, others have studied the issue, and it appears to hold up. An inescapable conclusion is that, going forward, the search for antisocial genes must take environmental factors into account.[13]

Other neurotransmitters must be involved with aggression, violence, and presumably ASP, but they have been much less studied. Dopamine is a prime candidate because of its role in mediating risky behaviors, as well as its role in the brain's reward system, which is why it is often referred to as the "pleasure neurotransmitter." Its role in aggressive behavior is based on circumstantial evidence that includes the fact that stimulant drugs—legal and illegal—rev up dopamine and can lead to impulsive violence. On the other hand, drugs that dampen dopamine drive (antipsychotic medications, for example) have been used to reduce hostility and aggression across a range of psychiatric illnesses, including schizophrenia and traumatic brain injuries. Experimental evidence for the role of dopamine has not always been consistent, but an early finding was that recidivist criminals (most of whom were antisocial) had *lower* levels of a chemical metabolite (or breakdown product) of dopamine called homovanillic acid, suggesting less dopamine turnover. Attention has now turned to variants of the dopamine receptor gene (there are several, and all are called *polymorphisms*). This work strongly suggests that traits associated with ASP (such as novelty-seeking and impulsivity) are associated with different dopamine receptor polymorphisms that are genetically transmitted.[14]

HORMONES AND DIET

Antisocial behavior has also been attributed to abnormal circulating levels of testosterone, the male hormone thought responsible for certain traits, including aggression. Like serotonin, testosterone and other male hormones probably developed in a primitive world where aggression was necessary to survival. High levels of testosterone have been associated with aggressive behavior in a wide range of animal species and, in humans, among violent prisoners. The link between antisocial behavior and male hormones—androgens—is supported by several lines of research. First, anti-androgenic medication (discussed more fully in Chapter 7) given to dangerous sex offenders to reduce their levels of male hormones has been shown to reduce violent sexual impulses. Second, research on male athletes who abuse anabolic steroids—synthetic male hormones—to improve performance and enhance muscle mass shows that these drugs can also fuel anger and aggressive outbursts. Several murders committed by athletes are reported to have occurred under the influence of anabolic steroids. Third, teenage boys with chronic antisocial behavior or disruptive behavior have higher circulating levels of androgens, including testosterone, as compared to boys without these behaviors.[15] The research is not conclusive, but indicates that excessive androgens may well influence the development or expression of violent and aggressive behaviors, at least in men.

Other chemical theories of antisocial behavior—and perhaps ASP—cast light on diet and the way the body reacts to substances found in food. Although hypoglycemia, or low blood sugar, has been the focus of dubious notions tying sugar to nearly every human ailment, legitimate researchers remain intrigued by the idea that it may influence behavior. Glucose levels of less than 80 mg per deciliter (the normal range is 80–110 mg/dL) can skew the brain's normal functions, producing anxiety, irritability, and aggression. Low blood sugar could even be a precipitating factor in some violent outbursts. Research has shown, for example, that prison assaults peak between 11 and 11:30 A.M., a period when symptoms of reactive hypoglycemia are also most common. More recently, a study of Boston high school students found a dose–response relationship between non–diet soft drink consumption and violence: the greater the consumption, the greater the propensity for violence. One possible explanation offered by the researchers was that low blood sugar produced by wildly fluctuating levels of sugar intake contributed to the violence.[16]

The link between low blood sugar and violence has led some researchers to claim that antisocial behavior can be modified through dietary changes. This claim is based on the observation that diets high in refined carbohydrates can lead to extreme variations in blood glucose levels. Because such foods are rapidly absorbed in the gut, they can produce an immediate rise in blood glucose. This, in turn, triggers a large secretion of insulin, which causes an overreduction in blood glucose. A two-year study of juvenile delinquents fed a diet low in refined carbohydrates observed a nearly 50% drop in disciplinary offenses.[17] Although the idea that manipulating one's diet might reduce antisocial tendencies remains controversial, perhaps some of us really are influenced by what we eat and drink.

DAMAGED BRAINS

Many scientists have conjectured that antisocials' central nervous systems are damaged, an idea first expressed in the mid-19th century by psychiatric pioneer Benjamin Rush, whose contributions are profiled in Chapter 2. Supporting evidence has accumulated since the 1940s, when the first crude electroencephalographic (EEG) tracings of brain wave activity revealed that abnormal patterns were two to three times more common among antisocials than among others.[18] Today, modern techniques like magnetic resonance imaging (MRI) and positron emission tomography (PET) scans provide detailed pictures of brain structure and activity, allowing researchers to link certain behaviors to different brain regions. Many, including myself, believe Rush was correct when he attributed chronic antisocial behavior to a brain dysfunction.

In simple terms, the brain has five interconnected regions. The most primitive area is the *brain stem*, which regulates basic body functions like breathing and blood pressure. The *diencephalon* is next, and is the seat of sleep and appetite. The *cerebellum*, an oval structure that adjoins the brain stem, controls equilibrium and movement. The *limbic system* forms a loop of structures that govern sexual behavior and instinctual emotions. Covering these structures is a thick layer of gray matter, known as the *cerebral cortex*, where sensory messages are received and thought is processed. A portion of the cortex located behind the forehead—the prefrontal lobes—serves to modulate the messages that surge within the brain, providing judgment, organizing behavior, and regulating decisions. The cortex and its frontal lobes are small and underdeveloped in lower species and are thus largely responsible for making us human. When these interrelated systems are thrown off balance, a variety of biological, behavioral, and cognitive problems can emerge.

Antisocials display many of the symptoms shown by patients who have suffered strokes or injuries to the prefrontal lobes. University of Southern California neurologists Antonio and Hannah Damasio, and others, have shown that damage to these regions can destroy the emotional—and perhaps moral—compass that controls behavior. In his book *Descartes' Error: Emotion, Reason, and the Human Brain,*

Antonio Damasio describes one of the most important cases in the annals of medical literature—important because it led to the observation that certain brain regions are dedicated to behavior, emotions, and reasoning.[19] During the summer of 1848, construction foreman Phineas Gage was grievously injured in a quarry accident in Cavendish, Vermont. Gage was using an iron rod to tamp down a mixture of explosive powder and sand in a rock ready for blasting. Distracted, he set off an accidental explosion that drove the rod through his skull. It entered the left cheek, pierced the base of the brain, shot through the frontal region, and exited the top of his head.

Although Gage miraculously survived the freak accident, he was never the same. Where there was once a responsible, industrious citizen, there was now a man described as "fitful, irreverent, indulging at times in the grossest profanity...impatient of restraint or advice...obstinate, yet capricious and vacillating." He lived for 13 years after the blast but moved frequently and was often fired from whatever work he could find. For a time, he was a featured attraction at Barnum's museum in New York, where he displayed his wounds and the 3-foot-7-inch, 13-pound rod responsible for his injuries.

Gage's case, Damasio writes, illustrates how damage to specific brain regions can disrupt "the personal and social dimensions of reasoning." He explains how Hanna Damasio, his wife and colleague, used MRI technology and Gage's preserved skull to create computer images of his brain, showing both the location and the extent of the damage.[20] When the rod passed through Gage's left and right prefrontal cortices, it destroyed an area responsible for rational decision making and the processing of emotion. This case and many others reported in the medical literature document the effect of similar brain injuries resulting from accidents, assaults, wartime combat, and prefrontal lobotomies for mental illness. For example, Vietnam veterans with significant injuries to the frontal lobes were two to six times as violent or aggressive as veterans who had not experienced such injuries. Because people with brain injuries or degenerative illnesses like Alzheimer disease can develop aggressive and impulsive behaviors that resemble ASP, they have been described as having "acquired sociopathy."[21]

Other clues suggesting brain injury in antisocials are circumstantial but highly intriguing.[22] Children with conduct disorder often have learning disabilities, especially trouble with listening, reading, problem solving, writing, and speaking, and this could indicate mild brain damage. Minor anomalies in facial appearance like a weak chin or low-set ears—sometimes thought to be observable markers of hidden neurodevelopmental defects—are unusually common in such children. In general, antisocials have lower average IQ scores than others, are more likely to be diagnosed as hyperactive while children, and more often have coexisting ADHD. None of these findings is especially important on its own. But taken together, they provide suggestive—although admittedly indirect—evidence of abnormal neurodevelopment. A wide range of factors can disrupt the central nervous system as it develops in the womb and in early life, creating a tendency for antisocial behavior. Poor prenatal nutrition, drug abuse and smoking by the pregnant mother, or birth complications that rob the child's brain of oxygen are among a few such factors identified through careful research.[23]

ARE THEY WIRED DIFFERENTLY?

Brain imaging is one of the most active areas of neuroscience research. Although no one has found the seat of antisocial behavior, the clear implication of this work is that the brains of antisocials and psychopaths—its more severe variant—are "wired" differently than others. The development of brain imaging methods took off in the 1970s, when computed tomographic (CT or CAT) scanning was introduced, but has accelerated along with the proliferation of newer techniques that provide better resolution of brain structure (for example, MRI) or methods that can be used to investigate brain function, including functional MRI and PET. The search is now on to assess connections between abnormal brain structure and function in antisocial (or psychopathic) individuals, and also to link behavioral traits like aggression or even pathological lying to particular brain regions.

In an early study, psychiatrist Peter Goyer and colleagues at the National Institute of Alcohol Abuse and Alcoholism used PET to assess brain function in Navy and Marine personnel who had assaulted others or made suicide attempts.[24] (PET is a computerized technique that uses radioactive substances, usually a form of glucose, to track the movement and rate of the brain's metabolism.) The most aggressive men showed striking changes—including impaired ability to process glucose, the primary energy source for working neurons and other cells—in the right temporal lobe, an important part of the limbic system that helps regulate mood and behavior. This was an early clue that the limbic loop was an important area for researchers to target.

Psychologist Adrian Raine, a leader in the quest to solve the mystery of antisocial behavior, and his colleagues have carried out a series of innovative studies to peer into the brains of antisocials and psychopaths.[25] Using PET to measure glucose uptake in murderers, Raine and his team found dramatic impairments in the prefrontal cortex and other underlying areas that make up part of the limbic system. An MRI study found that antisocial men had reduced gray matter volume in the prefrontal lobes, indicating for the first time that anomalies in this crucial brain structure may underlie at least some antisocial behavior. In an attempt to localize symptoms to a brain region, Raine's team next looked at a group of pathological liars, a common symptom in ASP, and, to their surprise, determined that liars had an *increase* in their prefrontal white matter. (White matter underlies the gray matter and relays and coordinates communication between brain regions.) They humorously compared this with "Pinocchio's nose" to suggest that repeated lying activates the prefrontal circuitry, leading to permanent changes in brain structure; like the nose that grew with repeated lies, so too does the psychopath's white matter! Raine's work continues, and, most recently, his team found smaller amygdala in psychopaths compared to controls. (The amygdala is a brain structure within the limbic system and is known to process fear and other emotions.) Raine and colleagues surmise that abnormally functioning amygdala lead to the psychopath's shallow emotions and derailed normal social development that contribute to callous and unfeeling behavior.

Kent Kiehl, who directs the MIND Research Network at the University of New Mexico, and who was strongly influenced by Robert Hare (who developed the Psychopathy Checklist), has also worked to unravel the mystery of antisocial and psychopathic behavior. Many of his imaging studies have used the technique called functional MRI to investigate brain activity in psychopaths during various emotional and cognitive experiments.[26] In their first study, Kiehl and colleagues reported reduced activity in the amygdala in psychopaths compared to controls in response to hearing emotionally charged words. As suggested earlier, a malfunctioning amygdala may keep children from learning to avoid behaviors with unwanted or bad outcomes, like hurting others, or from developing a normal conscience. A later study showed, under similar conditions and using a different experimental task, that psychopaths had *increased* activation in the right temporal lobe, a key region that had been identified by Goyer and colleagues in their study of military personnel. Kiehl and his team suggested that a malfunction in this brain area could contribute to the fearlessness that characterizes many psychopaths.

The work of Raine, Kiehl, and others is helping to close the loop in the search to understand the neural basis for antisocial and psychopathic behaviors. Even if imaging studies fail to identify their home, there is little doubt that subtle anomalies in brain structure or function underlie these conditions, and that specific brain regions are implicated, many within the limbic system that governs emotion and behavior.

NERVOUS SYSTEM QUIRKS

A large body of research has accumulated since the 1940s that suggests that antisocial and psychopathic behavior results from a strangely unresponsive nervous system rendering the person chronically underaroused and needing a "fix" of sensory input to produce normal brain function.[27] (*Psychophysiology* the area of research concerned with exploring connections between psychological functioning and physiological measures.) Much of the research has focused on samples of criminals, delinquents, or psychopaths—groups that overlap with ASP. Early studies found that EEG tracings of brain waves were abnormal in about half of those studied, showing the patterns of slow-wave activity more often seen in children and adolescents. Some researchers interpret this finding as evidence of brain immaturity, positing that a psychopaths' brain develops at unusually slow rates (although such EEG readings may also occur if subjects are drowsy or bored with the test). Men who repeatedly disrupt the lives of others without any semblance of empathy can indeed seem to be emotionally or morally stunted, lending this theory a certain intuitive appeal. A "maturational lag"—as yet unproved—could help explain the gradual improvement seen in some antisocials and offers one reason why violent crime tends to drop off when offenders reach their late 20s.

Delinquent children and psychopathic adults have repeatedly shown a low resting heart rate—the pace at which a heart beats under minimal demands, perhaps an indication of chronic underarousal.[28] This contrasts with the rapid pulse typically associated with anxiety and aroused states. Perhaps this accounts for Cleckley's observation that psychopaths do not experience anxiety. What he may have had in mind was that situations that provoke anxiety in most people, like telling a lie, committing a crime, or engaging in high-risk behaviors, don't affect psychopaths in the same way. This may be why some criminals appear cool and collected when presented with evidence of their misdeeds or why they are able to commit antisocial acts without any sign of anxiety, fear, or remorse.

Another psychophysiological measure that distinguishes psychopaths and criminals from others is skin conductance activity, the measure of current between two electrodes placed on the hand. Skin conductance at rest is quite low, but it increases the more one sweats, as with anxiety. When a neutral stimulus—like a particular sound—is followed by an aversive stimulus that boosts skin conductance—perhaps a mild electric shock—most people learn to link the two. Eventually, the sound alone will rouse the same degree of skin conductance as the shock itself. Psychopaths do not respond to such stimuli as others do, and their skin conductance remains low in situations that would elicit anxiety and increased conductance in normal individuals. This phenomenon may help explain British psychologist Hans Eysenck's observation that conscience stems from a set of classically conditioned negative emotional responses to situations associated with punishment.[29] Most of us develop a feeling of uneasiness at the mere contemplation of an antisocial act—possibly by linking such thoughts to negative repercussions. Perhaps the antisocial lacks this normal response pattern, explaining not only his failure to develop a conscience, but his tendency to seem inwardly calm in the face of external threats.

Yet another psychophysiological abnormality that marks psychopaths is the event-related potential (ERP)—tracings of brain waves that occur in response to an interesting stimulus. In psychopaths, the amplitude of these tracings tends to be greater than in normal people, usually following a brief delay. Adrian Raine theorizes that the initial delay represents baseline low arousal but that the subsequent boost in brain wave activity suggests enhanced attention to stimulating events.[30] He suggests that individuals with chronically low arousal seek out potentially dangerous or risky situations, like crime or violence, to raise their arousal to more optimal levels and satisfy their craving for excitement.

A fascinating study by Raine and his colleagues gives the theory of underarousal a boost.[31] They obtained EEG tracings and measures of resting heart rate and skin conductance from a group of 15-year-old English schoolchildren whom they monitored for nine years. Those who committed crimes were more likely to have had a low resting pulse at baseline, reduced skin conductance, and more slow-wave EEG activity than the others. Although Raine acknowledges that psychophysiological measures alone cannot explain criminal behavior, his results support the notion that at least some antisocial behavior may stem from subconscious efforts to jump start a chronically unresponsive nervous system.

FAMILY TIES

Ruben Deases, the young murderer profiled earlier in this chapter, grew up in a disturbed, violent home. His five brothers were delinquent. His alcoholic father regularly beat their mother. His paternal grandfather reportedly strangled a child to death. Rarely is an intergenerational cycle of antisocial behavior better documented. To some, the troubled Deases family only confirms the genetic transmission of antisocial symptoms. To others, it focuses attention on the role of family and home environment in shaping behavior. Wouldn't anyone, they ask, who grew up in such a family be emotionally scarred by the experience?

The current attention given to biochemical, physiological, and developmental causes of ASP overshadows a considerable body of evidence that points directly to the family and home environment as major contributors to antisocial behavior. Many children who become antisocial endure poverty, substandard housing, bad neighborhoods, parental abuse and neglect, and inadequate nutrition and medical care. Low socioeconomic level alone is probably not an important factor in delinquency, since poor children whose family lives are otherwise normal are unlikely to become antisocial.[32] But combined with other environmental hazards, being poor may become a risk factor in the development of ASP. It comes as no surprise that parents of troubled children show a high level of antisocial behavior themselves and that, in some cases, a chaotic home life and parental mismanagement can be traced to the disorder. The irony is that parents whose children are difficult to manage are often the least emotionally and financially able to cope constructively with behavior problems.

A study conducted in the 1940s by Sheldon and Eleanor Glueck, whose groundbreaking work is described in Chapter 5, was one of the first to show the connection between antisocial behavior and the family. The Gluecks compared 500 delinquent and 500 nondelinquent boys roughly matched for important characteristics like age and socioeconomic standing.[33] The parents of delinquent boys were more often alcoholic or criminal, and their homes were frequently broken by divorce, separation, or absence of a parent. Parents often were hostile and rejected their children, were inconsistent and erratic in their discipline, and were more likely to use physical punishment.

Later research confirmed the Gluecks' findings, prompting additional work to pinpoint those factors in the home most responsible for antisocial behavior. The most significant characteristic, some researchers learned, was the absence of one or both parents. Although prolonged separation from the mother was implicated by psychologist John Bowlby in his study of juvenile thieves, later studies found that the critical link was not the maternal bond, but instead the child's need to bond with *any* significant adult, regardless of that person's relationship with the child.[34] A grandparent, for example, could fill the role, so long as he or she provided an instructive model for interpersonal relationships. Depriving a young child of a significant emotional bond damages his ability to form intimate and trusting relationships later in life or to feel guilt when another person is wronged. This may be why some adoptees are prone to develop ASP. As young children, they may be more likely to move from one caregiver to another before a final adoption, thereby failing to develop appropriate emotional attachments to adult figures.

The impact of divorce or separation on a child's behavior depends on the initial quality of the parental relationship.[35] When parents cannot get along, their children may have little opportunity to observe normal affection and communication, and instead come to see fights and arguments as appropriate ways to solve disputes. In some instances, children may be better off after a separation or divorce, especially when the split saves them from a violent or abusive parent. Unhappy intact families probably produce more delinquency than relatively happy but broken homes. Remarriage is no panacea either, since many children have difficult and conflict-ridden relationships with stepparents.

Erratic or inappropriate discipline turns out to be one of the most important factors that influence antisocial behavior in children.[36] Antisocial or otherwise incompetent parents not only provide inconsistent discipline but also tend to rely on harsh punishment. Because inconsistent discipline rapidly becomes ineffective, parents escalate the intensity of punishment in an attempt to regain control. They alternate between permissiveness and harshness until discipline becomes irrelevant. If a child is verbally abused or beaten regardless of his behavior, the punishment loses its power and the child sees no advantage to being good. This may be why many antisocials do not seem affected by punishment or social sanctions and are unable to consider consequences unless they are immediate. As children, they never learned the connection between breaking the rules and paying the penalty.

Antisocial children also tend to be poorly supervised by their parents.[37] Involved parents carefully monitor their child's behavior, setting rules and seeing that they are obeyed, checking on the child's whereabouts, and steering him away from troubled playmates. Parents who provide good supervision take an interest in activities and schooling that help promote appropriate social behavior, making adequate parental supervision a vital component of a child's social development. Good supervision is less likely in broken homes because parents may not be available, and antisocial parents often lack the motivation to keep an eye on their children. The importance of parental supervision is also underscored when antisocials grow up in large families in which each child gets proportionately less attention. Large families themselves have been linked to delinquency, crime, and violence.[38]

After growing up in a disturbed home, some argue, the child enters the adult world emotionally injured. Without having developed strong bonds, he is self-absorbed and indifferent to others. Not having experienced consistent discipline, he has little regard for rules and little ability to delay gratification. Lacking appropriate role models, he learns to use aggression to solve disputes and fails to develop empathy and concern for those around him. In the end, he views society much the way he views his home and family—as a source of conflict rather than comfort. This is certainly true in the rants of killer Jack Abbott, whose story was told in Chapter 3, and who blamed society for creating the criminal he had become. Says Abbott: "When America can get angry because of the violence done to my life ... then there will be an end to violence, but not before."[39]

Several points need to be made about these theories of antisocial behavior. First, the fact that differences exist between the families of delinquents and nondelinquents does not mean that these variables cause antisocial behavior or ASP. Since the disorder seems to run in families, biological factors may be responsible for both problems in the home and misbehavior in the children who grow up there. Parents with a propensity for antisocial behavior do a poor job of raising children. The children themselves may inherit that same propensity, with their behavior influenced as much by genetics as by environmental factors. Delinquent children may be different from the outset, and thus elicit rejection and inconsistent punishment as a response to bad behavior rather than as a cause. Second, most researchers have treated delinquent children as a homogeneous group and have not taken into account various types of antisocial conduct. As we have learned from the work of psychologist Terrie Moffitt, the child whose delinquency begins in adolescence is probably much different from the child whose misbehavior was evident before school age.

BIRDS OF A FEATHER

A common observation made of troubled kids is that they often choose similar children as playmates, raising the possibility that negative peer influences contribute to antisocial behavior and help nurture conduct disorder and later ASP. Research shows that associating with delinquent peers increases a child's likelihood of delinquency. Sheldon and Eleanor Glueck found that 98% of delinquent boys had delinquent friends, which was true of only 8% of their nondelinquent counterparts.[40] This pattern of association (the "birds of a feather" phenomenon) usually develops during the elementary school years, when peer group acceptance and the need for belonging first become important. Aggressive children are among the most likely to be rejected by their peers, and this rejection drives social outcasts to form bonds with one another.[41] Socially rejected children tend to "hang out" together and form relationships that can encourage and reward aggression and other antisocial behaviors.

Another aspect showing the importance of peer relationships is the tendency for kids who admire antisocial peers to imitate their behavior. This phenomenon was portrayed in the popular film *The Christmas Story*, in the relationship between Scut, a large red-headed bully, and his smaller sidekick, Grover. Although Scut didn't think much of him, Grover helped Scut terrorize the other kids to gain his favor. This effect is apparently true *only* for kids not considered "cool" by their antisocial peer. The "uncool" youth engages in bad behavior—arguing, fighting, and bullying—to gain the acceptance of the antisocial peer.[42]

Early associations with delinquent children may later lead to gang membership. Gangs are especially attractive to children who feel ignored and neglected by their nondeliquent peers and family. Some gangs become substitute families for their members, imposing their own regulations. In her book *Do or Die*, journalist Leon Bing quotes a probation officer who describes the appeal of gang membership: "You feel wanted. You feel welcome. You feel important. And there is discipline and there are rules."[43] Many crime syndicates are well known for fostering a sense of belonging, for example, the Mafia "families" that ruled organized crime for decades, a group chillingly portrayed in the *Godfather* movies.

Does association with delinquents cause delinquency, or do antisocial traits prompt a child to associate with deviant peers? My own belief is that persons with a propensity for antisocial behavior seek out like-minded friends. Research has shown that children who are difficult before reaching school age—before they have an opportunity to associate with other similar children—are more likely to become delinquent than their better-behaved peers.[44] But peer influences alone are probably not sufficient to explain the worst cases of antisocial behavior in children, and other explanations likely come into play.

ABUSE AND ITS LASTING EFFECTS

Although child abuse has been implicated in everything from relationship problems to serial murder, its link to ASP makes it one of the more plausible environmental contributors to antisocial behavior. Antisocials are more likely than normal individuals to have histories of childhood abuse—not surprising, since many of them grew up with neglectful and sometimes violent antisocial parents.[45] In many cases, abuse becomes a learned behavior that formerly abused adults sadly perpetuate with their own children. But it also can carry physical effects that impact brain functions and create the route by which a brutalized child becomes a violent adult. Adrian Raine has reported findings from a study of 4,269 boys, many of whom suffered some form of birth complication and were raised by abusive mothers.[46] Those with histories of both birth complications and abuse were three times more likely than the others to be arrested for a violent crime by age 18. Raine has argued that early abuse, such as vigorously shaking a child, is especially harmful, because it can lacerate white matter nerve fibers that link the prefrontal cortex with deeper brain structures, areas that may be involved in generating aggressive impulses usually controlled by the prefrontal lobes. As we have learned, a functioning prefrontal cortex is crucial in controlling one's baser instincts.

The theory that abuse—physical, sexual, or even verbal—may actually change brain structure and function could be a key to understanding its lingering effects.[47] Brain development continues throughout childhood and into adolescence and is subject to environmental influence. In the developing brain, neurons in the cortex differentiate and make connections with other cells, forming the neural systems that underlie behavior. Traumatic events like abuse, according to this theory, can disrupt the wiring process and affect the brain's response to environmental stresses. By triggering a cascade of hormones and other brain chemicals, stressful events alter the patterns of neural development. Thus, abuse is one environmental factor that may change the anatomy and physiology of the brain, possibly resulting in some of the biological abnormalities linked to antisocial behavior.

THE ROLE OF MEDIA VIOLENCE

For many years, people have assumed that exposure to media violence is not only bad, but has the potential to unleash, or at a minimum, encourage antisocial behavior in those who view it. Television was the cause of violence, said its critics, who would point to the long hours that children—and their sedentary parents—would spend glued to the "tube." There has been a relentless increase in violent depictions since the introduction of television in the 1950s, to the present smorgasbord of viewing available in our homes 24/7 through multiple media outlets (including television and the Internet). Add to these the popular and violent video games that even our youngest children play, and it is no surprise that reasonable people have questioned whether there isn't something to this concern. This, combined with the near impossibility of parents' ability to consistently monitor their child's viewing (and gaming) preferences, gives one pause. Could the level of exposure to violence incite our children to commit heinous acts, such as school shootings that seem to come at a rapidly accelerating pace? Or could they fuel more mundane criminal acts, such as an assault, breaking and entering, or even vandalism?

Social scientist L. Rowell Huesmann and colleagues at the University of Michigan have extensively researched the issue, and they conclude that evidence is overwhelming and that "exposure to media violence does indeed relate to the development of violent behavior."[48] It is thought that kids become desensitized to violence and learn to accept a more hostile view of the world. The kids most vulnerable to this onslaught appear those who already live in a "culture of violence" in which there are few curbs against aggressive behavior—in other words, the homes that many antisocials grow up in.

NO SINGLE CAUSE

Let me retrace what we know about the causes of ASP, a disorder that appears to be determined by multiple factors. There is convincing evidence that ASP has a hereditary basis, and studies of twins and adopted children bolster what often has been observed informally: Crime, violence, turbulent lives and, ultimately, ASP tend to run in families. Current research suggests that the disorder's transmission from parent to child is due to something more than environmental influences, although the histories of abuse and deprivation common among antisocials indicate that biology and environment both play a role.

Both low levels of serotonin and high levels of testosterone have been associated with violent behavior, and it is possible that ASP reflects a chemical imbalance brought on by any number of hereditary and environmental causes. Other evidence, including brain scans of antisocials and psychopaths, suggests that malfunction in crucial brain regions is linked to bad behavior. Psychophysiological research has found that some antisocials have abnormalities of the nervous system that may influence behavior, perhaps by producing a chronic craving for stimulation.

A middle ground unites these varied observations and explanations. It is quite possible that different people arrive at ASP by different routes, and that those with a greater number of risk factors (or *hits*, a term that many researchers use) are more likely to develop the disorder. Some may have a genetic form of the illness, whereas others may develop it following mild brain injury during or shortly after birth. Still others may be affected by years of childhood abuse, neglect, or emotional deprivation. These propositions are not mutually exclusive, and it is possible to conceive of ASP as a condition that sprouts and flourishes in the right mix of circumstances. The genetic predisposition toward antisocial behavior and ASP may in fact manifest itself in different degrees. Perhaps those who inherit a more powerful genetic contribution develop the disorder regardless of circumstances, whereas those with milder genetic input require injury, deprivation, or abuse for ASP to result. Those with the weakest genetic element may exhibit only minor antisocial behaviors, or perhaps none at all. In this scenario, genetic makeup alone does not determine one's destiny.

Despite what we know about the long-term course of ASP, I prefer not to think of the disorder as a foregone conclusion for anyone. We do not know what causes it or how to prevent or cure it, but we do know that change is possible. Genetic and social forces may conspire to make people antisocial, but they do not necessarily doom them to remain so. For whatever reason, many antisocials improve and some remit. Perhaps we can learn from their example.

Chapter 7

Overcoming
Antisocial Personality Disorder

Options for Treatment

RUSS AT 49

Of all the men in my study, Russ was among the easiest to find. Sue Bell located a current address and telephone number in his hospital records and, when contacted, Russ readily consented to an interview at his home. He provided careful instructions to his house in Atlantic, a tidy Iowa town. Sue found the house just as he had described it—a two-story white and green structure in need of painting. The smell of fresh-cut grass drifted above the lawn, and the sound of a radio crackled through the house's screened windows.

Russ was waiting at the door and politely welcomed Sue into his home. She observed his slow walk and slight stoop, features offset by a boyish face and thatch of blond hair. His blue eyes, however, held a certain coldness that she found mildly unsettling. Inside, the house was neat but less than inviting, its living room furniture draped with bed sheets and its shag carpet worn with years of use. The frayed decor, with its dominant browns, oranges, and greens, suggested to Sue that the house had changed little since the 1970s. Still, she appreciated the absence of spent liquor bottles and assorted trash she had found in the homes of some study subjects. Russ directed them to the dining room table and offered her a seat, lowering the volume on the radio, which turned out to be a police scanner. After having had back surgery for a ruptured disc that left him partially disabled, one of his hobbies had become following police reports, Russ explained. He lit up an unfiltered cigarette—the first of many during the interview—and admitted that smoking ran contrary to his doctor's advice, especially since a heart attack two years earlier. Sue found Russ soft spoken and cooperative, a relatively easy man to interview.

In 1966, at age 28, Russ had been ordered to enter the University of Iowa's Psychopathic Hospital after a month's stay in the county jail awaiting trial on an aggravated-battery charge. He was accused of beating and stealing $90 from a man met in a bar, a brutal crime for which the courts demanded a psychiatric evaluation. "I'm here for a mental checkup," Russ had told the hospital's admitting physician upon arrival. He denied the incident that had led to his arrest and suggested it might have happened during an alcoholic blackout, although he acknowledged making a habit of bar fights and conceded that the beating could have happened.

His initial diagnosis was "sociopathic personality disturbance," but he remained sociable and forthcoming throughout the examination. The doctors described him as physically "well developed and well nourished." His fingers and arms carried crude tattoos reading "love," "mother," and "Russell." He showed no evidence of hallucinations or delusions, but the detachment with which he recalled his history of trouble concerned his admitting doctor. "He talked quite blandly about all of his difficulties and seems to have no guilt associated with this behavior," the doctor wrote. "He is at a loss to explain why he does these things, but openly admits he has no control over these impulses." For a week, Russ was carefully monitored by physicians and psychiatric ward personnel, who noted nothing unusual. His electroencephalogram (EEG) was normal, and extensive psychological tests brought no surprises. Eventually, he was discharged and returned to jail to await trial, leaving the hospital with a "guarded" prognosis and no recommendations for treatment—aside from the option of aversion therapy once his legal troubles were resolved, a treatment sometimes used back then to steer people away from alcohol.

Questioned by Sue, Russ recalled the hospitalization and the crime it had followed. The man he had beaten thought himself tough and needed a lesson—not unlike a lot of men encountered during his drinking days, Russ said with a chuckle. He had taken up alcohol during his early teens, a period of torment for his widowed, deaf mother. Aside from drinking anything he could get his hands on, Russ skipped school, defied her orders, and finally ended up in a boys' reformatory for a year. Upon his release, he enlisted in the Army, where he went AWOL and was kicked out after a court martial, an event he described with obvious shame. He became a temporary day laborer and moved from job to job, following the typically antisocial pattern of being fired or spontaneously quitting. His relationships were equally impermanent. He had been married three times, the first time at age 23. Recovering from a car accident, he fell for the nurse who took care of him, even though she was eight months pregnant by another man. At first, he thought the marriage might last. He adopted his wife's infant daughter and gave her his name, despite the objections of his in-laws. They had noticed what his wife had not, an escalating alcohol habit that left him shiftless and eventually abusive. She could take the arguing, the threats, and even the infidelity, but his physical assaults drove her from the home after four years. By then, they had three children, but Russ refused to support any of them.

Russ blamed alcohol for his life's problems and proudly told Sue that he had quit drinking at age 34, when he finally became, in his words, "sick and tired of being sick and tired." At his lowest point, he went from binge drinking to consuming up to a fifth of whiskey each day, falling into a state of regular blackouts and complete loss of self-control. He racked up nearly 100 alcohol-related criminal charges, the most serious of which sent him to a state prison for one year. Finally, after seven admissions to alcohol treatment programs, he managed to give up drinking. In his eyes, the achievement had changed everything. He told Sue that he had been married for 12 years and, with his wife, took in foster children, all of whom he told about his troubles with alcohol and the law with the hope that they would know him better and realize he could not be conned. His life was comfortable, and he was respected in the small community as a skilled machinist and active member of the Masons and Shriners—all admirable accomplishments, he noted, for a reformed felon. He owned several rental units and a vacation home in Arizona and socialized regularly at a nearby bingo parlor. His other hobbies included numerology, and he told Sue he believed his lucky number, 4, would help him win the next lottery jackpot. Growing older and wiser had helped him to settle down, he said, and he admitted being bothered by thoughts of people he might have hurt on his way to recovery.

MAKING THE CHANGE

Russ is a testament to what can happen when an antisocial finds the support—both internal and external—necessary to change his life. Although still relatively young (age 49) at follow-up, Russ was one of the men in my study who showed considerable progress. Clues to his attitude—the way he would smile when recalling his difficult days or how he hedged when admitting regrets—indicated that antisocial personality disorder (ASP) was still with him, perhaps shut away somewhere in his mind, ready to break free in the face of some unknown motivation. Certainly, information from a man who admits once telling "the wildest stories just to make people believe that I'm a great guy" should be taken cautiously, but I believe that much of the change Sue observed was genuine. A combination of factors, including health problems, a stable relationship, and recovery from alcoholism, likely contributed to his improvement. It is possible, too, that Russ had a somewhat mild case of ASP, although his family history (his father, brother, and sister all exhibited antisocial leanings) and personal record of misbehavior suggest otherwise.

Russ may seem like an odd example with which to open a chapter on treatment of ASP, as much of his improvement was mostly unrelated to therapy. He had never sought treatment for ASP, and his frequent hospitalizations for alcoholism were slow to bring results. Ultimately, change for Russ seemed to come from within, perhaps at a fortuitous time when he was poised for progress. The blend of personal motivation and circumstance is essential to any discussion of ASP treatment since there are no proven methods for overcoming the disorder. In fact, there has been little research into the treatment of ASP and almost no funding for such work. The word *treatment* may even have limited value when applied to ASP, because it suggests a patient who is suffering and seeking a cure. Most antisocials are not suffering in the usual sense. They may see no reason to abandon their ways and may even enjoy their escape from obligations, their impulsivity, and their freedom from guilt. Why seek out a normal life when it only seems to tie you down and restrict your options?

Faced with a steadfast refusal to seek help or even recognize the need for it, spouses, relatives, and friends caught in the web of ASP may surrender to hopelessness. The best they can expect is a gradual turn from crime and abuse, development of insight, and acceptance of responsibility—a distant prospect for many of those who face the daily challenge of living with an antisocial. The disturbing intensity of ASP at its worst gradually dims with time, but many family members are not able to wait. Fortunately, there are ways to cope with the disorder and even combat its effects. Once the diagnosis is made, family and friends must become allies in fighting ASP, as a sustained effort by all to break the antisocial patient's pattern of misbehavior is essential to changing the disorder's course.

OBSTACLE COURSE

The path to recovery has many obstacles. Looming largest is the infrequency with which ASP is diagnosed. Many mental health professionals fail to make the diagnosis even when the disorder is obvious. I believe that the stigma surrounding ASP and the therapeutic gloom that many associate with it keep some professionals from making the diagnosis. Instead, they—and their patients, too—remain focused on isolated manifestations of the disorder like temper outbursts, impulsivity, or recklessness rather than viewing them as parts of an overall pattern.

Another obstacle is the fact that few antisocials seek treatment, and their commitment to treatment is often lukewarm. Why should they change? To them, society and its tiresome standards are the problem. Of the men described in this book, very few sought treatment without coercion. Those like Russ, who seemed to recognize a need for change, are few and far between. In Russ's case, it was a frightening descent into alcoholism, including his frequent arrests and time in prison, that precipitated his effort to change. For some antisocials, threats of incarceration, loss of employment, or divorce illustrate the negative potential of the disorder and may drive them to seek help. For others, consistent pressure from family, friends, or the law may push them into treatment.

BEFORE TREATMENT

Because there are no standard treatments for ASP, it is essential to identify coexisting problems that *can* respond. A thorough evaluation like that described in Chapter 4 should confirm the diagnosis of ASP and seek evidence for accompanying depression, alcoholism or drug addiction, attention-deficit/hyperactivity disorder (ADHD), or other disorders. Treating coexisting disorders—depression, for instance, may respond to medication—can help reduce antisocial behaviors and prepare the person for the more complicated task of addressing ASP.

When an ASP diagnosis is made, it is important that the disorder and the diagnostic process be fully explained to the antisocial and any close family members. The diagnosis should be presented in a straightforward, nonjudgmental manner that does not minimize the potentially devastating nature of the disorder. The onus for improvement should be placed squarely on the antisocial's shoulders.

I've had many conversations over the years with antisocials, and they tend to go something like this: "Now that we've met to discuss your problems and your life, I've made some conclusions. Based on what you've told me, it's clear you've had lifelong difficulty getting along with others, dealing with authority, following rules and regulations, and controlling your temper. You might call this a *lifestyle disorder*, since it has affected every part of your life.

"Psychiatrists have developed a type of shorthand to explain problems and behaviors. This is a diagnosis. People with long-term difficulties like stormy relationships, job instability, or even criminal behavior have *antisocial personality disorder*. This doesn't mean that you don't like people. Instead, it means that you often find yourself at odds with society and don't like to follow its rules. This puts you in conflict with others and leads you, at times, to be your own worst enemy." At this point, I ask the patient about his feelings on what I've said, whether he thinks it is true. More often than not, the patient says something like "Yeah, you're right." Conversely, a few patients have told me to "take a flying leap" or something more colorful. Either way, my explanation continues:

"Let me tell you about ASP, since you probably haven't heard much about it. It starts early in life, usually in childhood, and is present by early adolescence. In its early phases, ASP causes problems at home and in school, like fighting with other children, lying to parents, or running away. Later problems include delinquency, alcohol and drug abuse, and problems on the job and in relationships. This may include trouble getting along with bosses or coworkers, getting to work on time, or getting work done. People with ASP may bicker and fight with their wives and partners, friends, and family members. All these problems can create serious consequences, alienating people with ASP from society and those around them. In the worst cases, antisocials become career criminals and end up in prison, have brief and troubled relationships, and have poor family ties.

"We don't know what causes ASP, but it may be something you were born with, and your home life while growing up may have had an influence. ASP is not something we can diagnose with blood tests or brain scans, and there are no pills for it, although medication can help with anger control and moodiness. Overcoming your antisocial tendencies involves hard work and effort, as well as marital and family counseling. By learning to overcome your symptoms, you can lead a happier and more productive life."

Some antisocials react strongly to this by becoming angry or defensive. Barring any real physical danger, this can be a positive sign, indicating that the diagnosis has hit a raw nerve and perhaps triggered a process of acknowledgment—the first step toward improvement. It may be helpful to show patients and their family members the diagnostic criteria in the American Psychiatric Association's *Diagnostic and Statistical Manual of Mental Disorders, Fourth Edition, Text Revision* (*DSM-IV-TR*) or to suggest additional reading, including this book. (A list of additional readings appears at the end of this book.) The next and most difficult step belongs entirely to the patient, for he must be willing to acknowledge the diagnosis and seek help.

ARRANGING TREATMENT

With the diagnosis confirmed and the person agreeing to seek help, the psychiatrist next develops a treatment plan. This may include medication but almost always involves talk therapy. Finding a knowledgeable and experienced therapist is essential. Although many psychiatrists are also psychotherapists, other mental health professionals—clinical psychologists, psychiatric social workers, and nurse clinicians—can also provide psychotherapy, often at a lower cost. The therapist needs to be familiar with community resources that can assist in recovery, including support groups, vocational guidance counselors, and other social services. He or she must also be accustomed to working with spouses, partners, and families, as their involvement is important.

Most psychiatric care takes place in outpatient settings, either private mental health practices or public clinics. Lower cost makes the latter a better option for many antisocials. Although some experts recommend highly structured, hospital-based inpatient programs for treating ASP, such therapy is expensive, and the programs have never been proven effective. For the most part, antisocials do not need the supervision afforded in psychiatric hospitals, where patients commonly include those at risk of harming themselves or others and those unable to care for themselves. Of course, the depressed, suicidal, violent, or addicted antisocial may need to be briefly hospitalized, but for others—the vast majority with ASP—hospital care is unnecessary.

Many experienced psychiatrists, myself included, are astonished that inpatient care is ever recommended for antisocials, other than for the few exceptions just noted. Antisocials can be a nuisance on inpatient units, becoming belligerent when their demands go unmet and using manipulation to gain their way, particularly as their days in the hospital drag on.[1] They can test the limits of both physicians and staff, often leaving abruptly after tumultuous stays. Tom, the first antisocial I treated, is a prime example of why inpatient treatment does not seem to work with antisocials. He flouted hospital rules, dominated discussions in group therapy, and made constant demands, to the point where all who worked with him were relieved when he left. I am convinced that Tom could have been better treated with a program of outpatient therapy, provided he adhered to its demands. Regardless of the setting, the potential success of therapy depends on the antisocial patient and his willingness to comply.

CHALLENGES

Treating antisocials in outpatient settings does not eliminate the problems they can cause therapists. They blame others, have a low tolerance for frustration, are impulsive, and have difficulty forming trusting relationships. They often lack motivation to improve and are notoriously poor self-observers. Antisocials simply do not see themselves as others do. It can be extraordinarily difficult to convince them that their self-image is distorted. Sessions may end abruptly if the patient is challenged or provoked, and the episode may end therapy altogether. A potential for violence lurks beneath the surface. At the same time, antisocials expect therapists to accommodate their demands and to be as interested in them as they are in themselves. Unrealistic about the goals of treatment, they may expect a quick solution to lifelong problems even while ignoring their therapists' recommendations. Sociologists William and Joan McCord, writing in 1956, compared these patients to a "chow dog who may turn and bite the hand that pets it," and describing therapy as a "thankless task."[2] Unfortunately, these observations remain true today.

Although trained to approach mental health problems in an objective, nonjudgmental, and goal-oriented way, therapists react with emotion as everyone else does, and treating antisocials can be a thorough test of one's professional resolve. *Countertransference* is a word used to describe therapists' emotional responses to their patients, whereas *transference* refers to the patients' feelings toward therapists. No matter how determined a therapist may be to help an antisocial patient, it is possible that the patient's criminal past, irresponsibility, and unpredictable tendency toward violence may render him thoroughly unlikable. Fortunately, it is not necessary to like a patient in order to help him. The effective therapist is aware of his or her own feelings and remains ever vigilant to prevent countertransference from disrupting therapy.[3]

A common emotional reaction among therapists toward antisocials is a feeling of fear, since stepping into an antisocial's life and challenging him to change makes us potential targets of violence. Patient assaults on therapists are actually quite rare, but they do happen, sometimes with grave results. In 1994, one of my former trainees, Tom Brigham, a talented and compassionate physician, was shot and killed in Spokane, Washington by an enraged patient upset that Tom had recommended his discharge from the Air Force. A psychologist who had reached the same conclusion also was killed. Although uncommon, murderous assaults like these may linger in the minds of fellow therapists. As well, feelings of helplessness and guilt may arise when therapy proves slow, difficult, or unproductive, particularly if one lacks experience with ASP. I know from my own experience as a young trainee how this reaction can cause a therapist to question his or her skills and profession. Although we learn in training that irresponsibility, lack of cooperation, and limited insight are aspects of ASP, the stubborn intransigence of many antisocials can come as a disheartening surprise. It is important that therapists confronting this reality for the first time understand their limitations and not lose sight of their professional identity and worth.

In extreme cases, therapists may experience feelings of rejection, anger, or even hatred in the face of their patient's seemingly immovable personality or record of misdeeds. A therapist may reject a patient in subtle ways—acting bored during therapy sessions or being late for appointments—or may ignore the patient altogether. The sense of revulsion that an antisocial's crimes or attitudes engender may cause therapists to question why they even bother to attempt treatment. Expressions of anger or irritation can occur before the therapist even realizes it. With the antisocial patient who enjoys testing his therapist's will and skills, such a reaction by the therapist can irrevocably sabotage treatment. With all this in mind, it is not surprising that many therapists prefer to have nothing to do with antisocials. The best prospects for treatment come with professionals well versed in ASP, able to anticipate their emotions and to present an attitude of acceptance without moralizing. They know their limits and have a sound sense of their professional identity. They are patient but firm in dealing with manipulation, and are willing to set limits. Last, they have abandoned rescue fantasies—notions like "Only I can save this patient"—recognizing that success depends more on the patient than on themselves.

APPROACHES TO THERAPY

Therapy for all manner of mental illnesses has a similar goal: to help the patient understand the nature and extent of his or her problems and encourage the person to make sensible changes. *Freudian psychotherapy* aims to uncover unconscious mental processes thought to motivate disturbed behavior. Psychiatrists since Cleckley have realized the futility of this approach, generally agreeing with his assessment that antisocials (the psychopaths of *Mask of Sanity*) do not change their behavior after psychoanalytic explorations of their unconscious minds. He wrote of patients treated for years with these methods who only "continued to behave as they had behaved in the past."[4] Most therapy is now less concerned with why behaviors developed than with how they can be eliminated, usually by changing the thinking patterns that lead to negative thoughts or actions. This emphasis on *cognitive behavioral therapy* (CBT) has largely replaced long-term therapy intent on mining the subconscious.

Cognitive behavioral therapy assumes that people develop inaccurate beliefs that trigger depression, anxiety, or behavior problems. A patient with depression, for instance, may wrongly believe that no one likes him, while another thinks her accelerated heart rate during a panic attack will lead to death. These false beliefs are *cognitive distortions* that the therapist will attempt systematically to challenge and correct, prompting the depressed patient to see that he is not friendless or the anxious patient to understand that she is healthy. In cases of mild depression and panic disorder, CBT techniques can be quite effective. One of the method's founders, psychiatrist Aaron Beck, has applied these therapy techniques to ASP and other personality disorders. Along with his colleagues, in the second edition of *Cognitive Therapy of Personality Disorders*, Beck describes the approach "as improving moral and social behavior through enhancement of cognitive functioning."[5] Cognitive behavioral therapy can be seen as a tool to correct or compensate for what is essentially faulty wiring in the antisocial brain, enhancing mental functions and reducing bad behavior. The goal is to help the antisocial patient make better moral decisions and halt his self-destructive tendencies.

Beck and colleagues have made several recommendations for applying this technique to ASP. First, the therapist should explain the treatment as a series of meetings and remind the patient that ASP is a serious problem that disrupts judgment and behavior, bringing long-term consequences. The patient is informed that treatment takes time and that any disadvantages will be far less severe than the possible repercussions of untreated ASP. The therapist should set guidelines for the patient's involvement in treatment, including regular attendance, active participation, and completion of any necessary homework outside office visits. If the patient fails to keep up his end of the bargain, becoming disengaged, hostile, or late for appointments, the therapist should confront him and review his choices. The patient must then decide whether to continue therapy, understanding that progress will require adherence to established guidelines. Therapy should proceed only when the patient benefits, not when his participation is marginal. A patient who submits to therapy only to avoid incarceration is not intent on improving, says Beck, and therapy must be more than a means by which an antisocial escapes the consequences of his behavior.

The cognitive behavioral model for treating the antisocial focuses on evaluating situations in which his distorted beliefs and attitudes interfere with functioning or achieving success. For example, an antisocial's explosive temper creates problems on the job when it causes him to be fired or limits his advancement. Unable to assess his actions critically, he may attribute a history of work conflicts to unjust persecution or other factors beyond his control, never pausing to examine the consequences of his actions. A major goal of therapy is to help the antisocial to understand how he creates his own problems, and how distorted perceptions prevent him from seeing himself the way others do. This can be delicate ground for a therapist to tread, and it is important that the antisocial not be coerced or shamed into admitting problems. Accusations will not convince him of the error of his ways, but rather may subvert the rapport between therapist and patient, and ultimately backfire.

Working together, patient and therapist develop a problem list—the more specific, the better. A patient who has trouble with uncontrolled aggression may be asked to identify situations in which this symptom rears its head, listing statements like "I yell at my wife when we argue." The list helps clarify problems and expose tensions, showing how and when they interfere with daily life. Once the problems are identified, cognitive distortions that underlie each of them are exposed and challenged. Typically, the antisocial has an extensive repertoire of mistaken beliefs that maintain and reinforce his behavior.

Some of the distortions most common to ASP, as outlined by Beck and colleagues, include *justification*, or the patient's belief that his desires are adequate grounds for his actions; *thinking is believing*, a tendency to assume that his thoughts and feelings are correct simply because they occur to him; *personal infallibility*, the idea that he can do no wrong; *feelings make facts*, the conviction that his decisions are always right when they feel good; *the impotence of others*, a belief that everyone else's views are irrelevant unless they directly affect the patient's immediate circumstances; and *low-impact consequences*, the notion that the results of his behaviors will not affect him. These self-serving beliefs share an emphasis on the antisocial's immediate personal gratification over eventual results, as well as a disturbing lack of concern about how his actions affect others. Like a child too young to have learned appropriate social behavior, he attempts to satisfy his desires without regard for anyone else. When his immediate wants go unmet or when others react in opposition to his behavior, the antisocial feels frustrated, angry, or impotent and may act out in response. The cognitive distortions that characterize ASP form the most difficult barrier to treating the disorder—the fact that few antisocials are willing or able to take even the first step toward questioning their behavior and attempting change.

Psychologist Robert Hare takes a dim view of therapy with psychopaths, those at the severe end of the antisocial spectrum, as discussed in Chapter 2. In offering an unvarnished view of therapy, he describes psychopaths as "well satisfied with themselves and with their inner landscape, bleak as it may seem to outsiders....Given these attitudes, it is not surprising that the purpose of [psychotherapy] is lost on psychopaths."[6]

Although therapy may not help those at the extreme end of the antisocial spectrum, what about those who constitute the majority of people with ASP? Beck and colleagues point out that antisocials are unfairly labeled as unable to profit from therapy, which they call the "untreatability myth." My own view is that because these myths have circulated among those in my profession for so long, they have prevented the field from moving forward to develop and refine effective treatments for ASP. I am not willing to write the antisocial off as treatment resistant or treatment refractory, or for being unworthy of treatment. Perhaps extreme cases *are* deeply ingrained, so rooted in basic brain functions that they stubbornly resist change, but therapy may, at the very least, provide an avenue by which some antisocials can learn to understand themselves and their disorder. This ought to be our focus.

There is no need to sugarcoat the challenges that treatment present. It is hard to overstate how difficult it can be to convince an antisocial that he might be at fault for his own problems and that the key to living a better life is a change of attitude. Yet CBT offers a sensible approach to help many antisocials develop the capacity to make appropriate decisions and get their lives on track. Kate Davidson, a psychiatrist at the University of Glasgow in Scotland, has taken up the challenge of refining the treatment for antisocials. She recently led a small scale study in which 52 antisocial men were assigned to CBT or "usual care" (meaning essentially anything other than CBT). Says Davidson: "The view from the ground...was that doing [CBT] was helpful in reducing antisocial behaviours and changing thinking." Although this (and other early data) suggests that the method can be helpful, only larger and longer term studies will reveal its true effectiveness.[7]

Glen O. Gabbard, a psychiatrist at Baylor College of Medicine, has outlined a set of "fundamentals" for engaging the antisocial. First, the therapist should be "stable, persistent, and incorruptible." Next, the patient's minimization of his antisocial behavior should be confronted and an attempt made to connect his behavior with his emotions; coexisting conditions—such as depression or alcoholism—should be addressed, as well as situational factors that may worsen his behaviors. Third, countertransference should be monitored to ensure that the therapist maintains perspective. Factors that do not bode well, says Gabbard, include any indication that the patient is at the psychopathic end of the antisocial spectrum, such as a history of sadistic violence, complete absence of remorse, or incapacity to develop emotional attachments; and either an IQ suggesting intellectual disability or an IQ in the superior range (because a low IQ may preclude full participation in the therapy, whereas a high IQ may lead to inappropriate intellectualizing and questioning of the treatment). Finally, he notes the "chill of dread." That is, a fear of predation experienced by the therapist is a sure sign of the presence of a malevolent, antisocial personality.[8] As one of psychiatry's leading lights, Gabbard's advice is worth considering.

WHAT ABOUT MEDICATION?

By some accounts, psychiatry is in the midst of a pharmacological revolution as new drugs designed to correct abnormalities in brain chemistry are prescribed for problems ranging from major depression to compulsive gambling. Much of the hype—and some of it is just that—surrounds a new generation of antidepressant medications called *selective serotonin reuptake inhibitors* (SSRIs), to which some patients and physicians attribute life-changing effects. These and practically every other drug that targets the central nervous system have been used to treat antisocials, but no medications are routinely used or specifically approved for ASP. Only a single drug therapy study has targeted antisocials, and this lack of research has been a serious impediment to making evidence-based recommendations for ASP. At present, there is no single pill that one can take to counter anger, habitual conning, persistent failure to accept responsibility, or lack of remorse all at once. Even if there were, the patient would have to be willing to take it.[9] Effective treatments require cooperation, patience, and compliance—low priorities for many antisocials.

That said, several drugs have been shown to reduce aggression, the chief problem for many antisocials. The best documented is lithium carbonate, which was found to reduce anger, threatening behavior, and assaults among prisoners studied in the 1960s and 1970s. The drug has also been shown to reduce behaviors like bullying, fighting, and temper outbursts in aggressive children. Phenytoin (Dilantin), an anticonvulsant, also has been shown to reduce impulsive aggression in prison settings.[10] Other drugs have been used to treat aggression in brain-injured, intellectually challenged, or psychotic persons, or in persons with borderline personality disorder. They include carbamazepine (Tegretol), sodium valproate (Depakote), and lamotrigine (Lamictal), all anticonvulsants; propranolol (Inderal), a blood pressure medication; buspirone (BuSpar), an antianxiety drug; and trazodone (Desyrel), an antidepressant.[11] Results are decidedly mixed. Although some aggressive patients seem to respond to medication—symptoms are reduced but not necessarily eliminated—many show little improvement.

Antipsychotic drugs, including haloperidol (Haldol), chlorpromazine (Thorazine), or risperidone (Risperdal), have also been studied in varied populations, including children with severe disruptive behaviors. Although these drugs may deter aggression, side effects limit their acceptability.[12] The older drugs, such as Haldol, can induce the potentially irreversible condition *tardive dyskinesia*, which causes abnormal movements of the mouth and tongue, while the newer drugs, such as Risperdal, can cause weight gain and metabolic issues, such as prediabetes, thus making them poor candidates for long-term use. Tranquilizers from the benzodiazepine class, including diazepam (Valium), clonazepam (Klonopin), alprazolam (Xanax), and lorazepam (Ativan), are not recommended in treating antisocials, because they are potentially addictive and may paradoxically lead the antisocial to act out on his impulses.[13]

Medication can help alleviate coexisting disorders such as major depression, panic disorder, or ADHD, producing a ripple effect that reduces antisocial behavior even in the absence of therapy that specifically targets ASP. This underscores the need for a thorough psychiatric assessment. Mood disorders are some of the most common conditions accompanying ASP and are also among the most treatable. More than two dozen drugs are available to fight depression, including the SSRIs. These medications, which include fluoxetine (Prozac), paroxetine (Paxil), sertraline (Zoloft), and citalopram (Celexa), are superior to their predecessors—the older tricyclic antidepressants and monoamine oxidase (MAO) inhibitors—because they are generally well tolerated and are safer in overdose. For reasons that remain unknown, depressed patients with severe personality disorders—including ASP—tend not to respond as well to antidepressant medication as other depressed patients, an observation that in itself should not prevent psychiatrists from prescribing these drugs.[14]

The SSRIs also have been used to treat aggressive behavior, based on the link between serotonin and aggression described in the previous chapter.[15] The drugs boost levels of serotonin in the central nervous system and, in theory, make up for the serotonin deficit associated with aggression and violence. Although SSRIs are probably no better at treating aggression than more traditional antidepressants, there is no evidence that they worsen violent tendencies, as has been alleged.

Other drugs studied as treatments for aggression may be useful in antisocials with bipolar (manic-depressive) disorder characterized by extreme mood swings. Lithium carbonate, carbamazepine, sodium valproate, and lamotrigine are effective in stabilizing mood swings in these patients, reducing both the highs and lows.

Stimulant medications paradoxically reduce symptoms of ADHD, a condition that can compound the aggression and impulsivity that accompany ASP. Methylphenidate (Ritalin) and dextroamphetamine (Dexedrine) are two of the most common medications used to reduce excessive activity, distraction, and attention problems in ADHD, although they should not be prescribed to patients with histories of drug abuse. Nonstimulant medications are available and have less abuse potential, including bupropion (Wellbutrin), atomoxetine (Strattera), and guanfacine (Tenex).

For those with dangerous and uncontrollable sexual behavior, injections of medroxyprogesterone acetate (Depo-Provera), a synthetic hormone that reduces circulating levels of testosterone, can be administered.[16] Given weekly or biweekly to cut sexual desire, it is usually well tolerated, although not entirely without side effects. Although its use is relatively uncommon, and it is not approved to treat these conditions, as an off-label remedy the drug offers a way to reduce the menace of repeat sex offenders, some of whom are antisocial.

CONFRONTING ADDICTION

Medication can relieve some of the mental health problems that tend to coexist with ASP, but other disorders require different approaches. In many antisocials, alcoholism and drug addiction are major barriers to treatment for the underlying ASP. These patients need help with their addictions before CBT or other approaches can succeed. Although abstinence from drugs or alcohol does not itself guarantee a reduction in antisocial behaviors, it is an essential first step, and it may be the reason why Russ, whose story was told earlier in the chapter, had improved.

Many mental health professionals regard substance abuse as a complex problem for which treatment often fails, but a carefully designed rehabilitation program—whether in a hospital or occurring in an outpatient setting—can succeed. Those who succeed tend to be the ones with the most to lose: good jobs, money and position, sound marriages, or supportive families. Because many antisocials lack these motivating factors, their treatment outcomes generally are not as good, but some, like Russ, come to realize the power of their addiction and successfully leave it behind. Research confirms that antisocial substance abusers who stop using alcohol and drugs are less likely to engage in criminal activity and have fewer family conflicts and emotional problems than before.[17]

Alcoholism and drug addiction, like ASP, are lifelong problems, and the antisocial patient must be reminded that recovery is an ongoing process. Following an inpatient or outpatient treatment program, the patient should be encouraged to attend meetings of an organization like Alcoholics Anonymous, the well-known program that, since 1935, has helped millions maintain sobriety with the support of fellow alcoholics. A key tenet of this program holds that addiction is overpowering but that behavior can be controlled. Obviously, this admission challenges the antisocial's ingrained notions of infallibility and superiority, as well as his lack of self-control. An alcoholic antisocial makes a valuable leap when he accepts the reality of his addiction, and this may bring him closer to applying the same insight to his ASP. Alcoholics Anonymous chapters, as well as those of sister organizations like Narcotics Anonymous and Cocaine Addicts Anonymous, exist throughout the country and should be recommended by therapists when appropriate.

Compulsive (pathological) gambling is another addictive behavior common in antisocials. Problem gamblers share many traits with alcoholics and other addicts, gradually increasing the amount of money they spend and experiencing withdrawal-like symptoms when deprived of their favorite pastime. The number of formal treatment programs has increased in the past decade, particularly as many states with legalized gambling have provided funding, as is true for Iowa. Gamblers Anonymous, an organization patterned after Alcoholics Anonymous, has chapters in many parts of the country, and the possibility of using medication to combat the problem is being actively investigated.

THERAPY WITH PARTNERS AND FAMILIES

For those antisocials whose partners and families accompany them in the downward spiral of ASP, marital and family counseling becomes an important part of treatment. Bringing family members into the process may help the antisocial patient realize the impact of his disorder, as others can back up what the therapist has to say and counter the patient's denials. Therapists who specialize in family counseling are often enlisted to address the antisocial's trouble maintaining an enduring attachment to his spouse or partner, his inability to be an effective parent, his problems with honesty and responsibility, and the anger and hostility that can lead to domestic violence. Antisocials who were poorly parented themselves may need special help to learn appropriate skills. (By law, any evidence of ongoing child abuse that emerges during therapy must be reported to state social service agencies.)

These sessions may be as important for family members as they are for the antisocial patient, helping them deal with the pain, guilt, and confusion that so many experience. The sessions also help convince family members that they must stop protecting the antisocial, as this only enables him to continue his cycle of misbehavior. The antisocial can dupe his family members, showing them only what he wants them to see. They must regain a sense that they are in control of their lives, something that often seeps away over years of living with ASP. They must also become allies in treatment, learning how they can help and steadfastly demanding that their antisocial relative attempt to change.

Writing about Alcoholics Anonymous or family counseling programs, I am reminded of how few antisocials actually make it this far. The antisocial man who enters therapy with the motivation to get better is unusual. All the options I have mentioned are possibilities, but there are no guarantees in treating ASP. With some antisocials, the best we can do is to keep them at a distance.

PRISON PROGRAMS

Incarceration may be the best way to control the most severe and persistent cases of ASP.[18] Keeping antisocial offenders behind bars during their most active periods of criminality would, at least in theory, reduce the social impact of their symptoms. However, incarceration is permissible only when antisocials violate the law and pass through the criminal justice system. Although traditional rehabilitation has not been very successful, therapeutic prison programs might help deter some criminals—including antisocials—from returning to crime.[19] These programs may include CBT, treatment for drug and alcohol problems or coexisting mental disorders, and family therapy or marital counseling when appropriate. They must also be flexible enough to accommodate additional priorities, like job training and education. Ongoing evaluation is essential to ensure these programs meet expectations.

PREVENTION

As with any other disorder, the best option for dealing with ASP would be to prevent it from developing in the first place. A truly effective prevention strategy would require knowing more about what causes the disorder. Although we know, for instance, that infectious diseases can be countered by halting the spread of pathogenic microbes—through vaccines, awareness campaigns, or measures like safer sex—preventing mental illness is a different matter. Even if we were to learn tomorrow the ultimate cause of ASP, prevention would be much more complex than giving an injection. Although we have yet to identify its causes definitively, we have learned enough about ASP risk factors and its natural history to know where prevention might begin. A comprehensive discussion of preventive strategies aimed at troubled kids is beyond the scope of this book, but any sound program is likely to include several basic components.

First, prevention efforts should target those at greatest risk for ASP—namely, children with conduct disorder. Parents and educators must understand that in every community there is a small minority of children whose abnormal personalities make them especially difficult to reach. Children without conduct disorder so rarely become antisocial that interventions targeting them are largely a wasted effort. Preventive measures must include both troubled kids and their parents. Therapy should teach children how to recognize and reject bad behavior, how to make acceptable judgments between right and wrong, and how to connect actions with consequences. Parents need special training that shows them how to identify and correct misbehavior as it occurs and how to steer their children away from negative influences like delinquent peers. Antiviolence programs—like one in the New York City public schools that uses peer mediation and other strategies to teach conflict resolution—also may help children find alternatives to lashing out. The New York curriculum includes a pilot program targeting children who show early warning signs of delinquency.[20]

One well-known attempt at prevention, the Cambridge-Somerville study, shows just how difficult it can be to reform misbehaving kids and deter them from further trouble. Described by William and Joan McCord in their book *Origins of Crime*, the study was conducted in the 1930s and 1940s, and involved 320 troubled boys who received intensive counseling and family therapy for up to eight years.[21] At first, about 20% of the test subjects appeared more improved than a control group, but the benefits seemed to fade over time. At follow-up many years later, the test subjects and those in the control group were doing roughly the same. The famed study has been criticized, mainly because of the high number of dropouts, which can compromise the quality of data collected.

What about those who have already transgressed? At a conference sponsored by the National Institute of Mental Health, Psychologist Mark Lipsey of Vanderbilt University summarized data on the effect of treating delinquents.[22] He concluded that although the benefits of treatment programs for juvenile offenders are modest, recidivism rates were 10% lower for those who went through treatment. The most successful programs were more structured and specific, emphasizing behavior modification or skills training. The least successful involved traditional counseling and deterrence strategies like "shock" incarceration—which gives young offenders stiff sentences that are later reduced to spur improvement. Other efforts to frighten delinquents into reforming, like the program profiled in the 1979 television documentary *Scared Straight*, have had poor results. In that documentary, troubled kids toured prisons and met inmates in an attempt to frighten them out of crime. In one study, delinquent kids who participated actually committed more crimes during a six-month period following the program than did a control group of delinquents who had not participated.[23] Likewise, despite their popularity, there is little evidence that *wilderness programs*—whereby delinquent kids are sent to camps that emphasize back-to-nature experiences where they learn to bond with and trust others—have any lasting impact.

Although attempts to shock delinquents out of misbehavior may fail or even backfire, this does not mean that strict and fair punishment of young offenders is ineffective. Waln Brown, a sociologist with the William Gladden Foundation, who himself had a conduct disorder, believes that juveniles who are apprehended, prosecuted, and punished for their first offenses are less likely to have adult convictions than are those who escape penalties.[24] His concept runs counter to a long-held sentiment in juvenile justice that labeling children criminals while young creates a self-fulfilling prophecy, causing them to spin out of control. I am inclined to agree with Brown. I don't believe children with real personality disturbances somehow will be encouraged to act out by being labeled. They are just as likely, perhaps more so, to continue their behavior if they are excused. This view of punishment for young offenders is consistent with Lee Robins's observation that the antisocial men she studied tended to do better in the long run if they had served short jail sentences earlier in life.

RUSS: THE ASSESSMENT

Although he had clearly improved, Russ displayed the marks of ASP, alcoholism, and life on the edge. He had deteriorated physically and showed signs of impaired memory and concentration, shortcomings that seemed to make him uncomfortable. Sue asked him to count backward from 100 by 7s. He quit after reaching 93. He was unable to spell the word *world* backward and had an exceedingly poor vocabulary, having to ask Sue the meaning of the word *abdominal*. Despite such problems, Russ had found a modicum of success in work, community life, and marriage—not quite normal, but much better off than many of his fellow study subjects. He showed no overt antisocial behavior, had given up drinking, and took responsibility for his foster children. In short, he was no longer a threat or burden to society.

Nevertheless, Sue and I felt that he showed lingering signs of ASP, which is not uncommon even among antisocials who have improved. He seemed to have few real regrets about his past, despite expressing a vague sense of guilt toward those he had hurt. In fact, he appeared a bit nostalgic when recalling the assault charge that had motivated his hospitalization years before. I was also struck by his complete loss of contact with his three biological children.

Perhaps antisocials never completely recover, always carrying with them vestiges of their personality disturbance. For some, improvement is a natural product of the aging process rather than a conscious goal, lending their past misbehavior the nostalgic flavor of youth. Even some of those patients who show the greatest change seem unable to comprehend the degree to which their actions affected those around them. They may continue to live in emotional isolation. Self-interest is a natural component of the human makeup, but it is especially strong in antisocials, and it leaves many of them unable to develop fully compassion, conscience, and other attributes that make for successful social relations. However, some antisocials manage to succeed by certain measures, acquiring wealth and prestige. For some, ASP may even provide the tools to realize their fantasies of power and superiority. Looking at the examples of antisocial men that I have offered so far, one might suspect that ASP inevitably means poverty and assorted other ills. But if antisocials are born, they are born into families of every class and neighborhood. If they are made, they sometimes end up the envy of those around them, seemingly accomplished men whose disorder remains mostly concealed. These are the men I take up in the next chapter.

Chapter 8

Power and Pretense

The Hidden Antisocials

HIDING IN PLAIN SIGHT

They start out as boisterous young toughs, driven by yearnings for excitement, rebellion, and intoxication, crippled by failure at school and work, damned by a lack of conscience and responsibility. They end up mired in addiction, poverty, and despair, having wrecked not only their own lives, but sometimes also the lives of others—partners, parents, children—unfortunate enough to have been dragged along. This is a common outcome of antisocial personality disorder (ASP), one that many people recognize among men they know. There is the cousin who dropped out of sight and could be in jail, the neighbor on perpetual disability who nurses beers in his backyard and bullies his wife, the homeless man who curses and begs from a favorite park bench. Battered into misery by their own misbehavior, these men seem to have no interest in what many people prize—relatively content, fulfilling, and productive lives.

Not all antisocials fit this picture, however. Antisocial personality disorder can appear in the closest families, the most comfortable neighborhoods, and the most highly regarded professions. Some antisocials manage to attain success despite their disorder. It is wrong to regard ASP as a disorder of the poor, even though poverty is a lifelong condition or an eventual outcome for many whom it affects. An antisocial's natural tendency to spurn authority, rules, and any concern for his future cuts him off from the goals of work and economic progress, and poverty is more likely an effect than a cause of the disorder (although growing up in deprivation may be one factor that triggers an underlying predisposition to ASP).

Like ASP, poverty is a condition that tends to pass from generation to generation, leaving many antisocials—as well as their normal relatives—caught in its trap. Conversely, an antisocial born into wealth may inherit the means to disguise his disorder. Protected from failure by a cushion of money and a veneer of respectability, he can evade the constraints of authority through the misguided assistance of family members, the aid of high-paid lawyers, and the shelter of private education. As long as the money lasts, he will probably be free to indulge his impulses without the everyday challenges that plague poorer antisocials.

Some antisocials manage to make their way through school and into the workforce, even becoming attorneys, businessmen, politicians, or other professionals. Many of these men come from economic circumstances that pave their way to success, giving them repeated opportunities to overcome errors of judgment and lapses into misbehavior. The character of ASP varies with the individual, and some are able to apply their intelligence to respectable ends. Others make up for a lack of initiative with sheer guile and charm, becoming successful con men otherwise indistinguishable from their neighbors. For some, ASP can be highly lucrative, as it lends them a talent for bilking a living from others, sometimes legally but often not. Others marry into money, take up the drug trade, or find other means to beat the odds and attain a comfortable existence. Later in this chapter, I will tell the story of Richard, a subject in my study whose ASP never remitted but who somehow managed to hide behind a quiet façade of suburban life. I was never able to determine exactly how he did it.

Money, it sometimes seems, can make a big difference in both how antisocial behavior is expressed and how it is viewed. Petty crime—vandalism, shoplifting, minor burglaries—may be interpreted in far different ways, depending on whether it is perpetrated by suburban kids or by young people from the inner city. Assumptions about class and wealth can lead people to see such infractions as youthful rebellion in one case, the onset of a career criminal in the other. Likewise, views of crime are tempered by the nature of the offense in question, making charges of fraud, embezzlement, and similar white-collar crimes seem more excusable than other violations, even though they all constitute antisocial behavior. To some extent, this disparity of attitudes carries over to more severe cases of antisocial behavior and even ASP. When a brutal act of violence takes place in a well-to-do community, or a criminal is found living in that same community, a common response is shock that "something like this could have happened here." Friends and neighbors remark that the offender seemed "so normal."

Think of the reaction of neighbors when former Boston crime boss Whitey Bulger—who had spent years on the FBI's most wanted list—was apprehended in 2011, after hiding out in a modest Santa Monica apartment for 16 years.[1] A troublemaker from early life, Bulger's criminal career included robberies, illegal gambling, loan sharking, and murder, eventually elevating him to leadership of the notorious Winter Hill Gang. Even a prison term at Alcatraz failed to stop his descent into crime. A sometime FBI informant, Bulger and his girlfriend fled Boston after learning he was to be arrested. Living under assumed names, the two disappeared into the diverse California community. Although neighbors found them a bit reclusive, several expressed shock to learn that their quiet complex was harboring a vicious killer. Said one, "I'm not quite processing it all quite yet."

In fact, such men are often far different from their nonantisocial peers, their external normality hiding deep turmoil. Antisocial behavior and ASP have no respect for boundaries, whether geographic, social, or economic, but cultural biases may make it more difficult to recognize and confront the disorder when it occurs in certain environments.

Psychiatrists are not immune to these dangerous, although not wholly unfounded, biases. Most patients with ASP have trouble maintaining work or making ends meet, and it often takes significant problems like the loss of a job, an arrest, or a debilitating addiction to make the disorder known. Those who hide their disorder beneath a veneer of success are sometimes described as *high functioning*, meaning that their ASP seems to have limited impact on their ability to get by in the world. This term has obvious limitations, as it may seem to elevate economic or career accomplishments over other potential symptoms like relationship problems, persistent lying, and a penchant for manipulation. Nevertheless, it reflects that fact that, in our society, money and status can effectively disguise ugly and destructive behaviors.

FAMILY VALUES

Years of working with antisocials and their relatives led me to question whether Leo Tolstoy's observation that "all happy families resemble one another; every unhappy family is unhappy in its own way" can be applied to ASP.[2] Although the torment and despair that stem from the disorder vary from situation to situation, I have seen many families react to the disorder in a similar manner, often rushing to the defense of an antisocial relative. The impulse to protect an antisocial member comes naturally to families, and lack of knowledge about ASP leads parents, spouses, and children to hope that their son, husband, or child has a short-term problem that they can correct. This reaction can have a particularly strong impact in families that possess the resources—emotional as well as financial—to keep bailing out their antisocial loved one. Although they may spare no expense on therapy and other efforts to break the pattern of misbehavior, their ultimate goal often is to protect the antisocial from legal trouble, even though sanctions may be what he needs to understand the danger of his ways. It can be difficult to persuade family members that coddling an antisocial only feeds his misbehavior, particularly when they have invested years of secrecy and sacrifice in doing exactly that. Fortunately, some families learn this on their own. Others may recognize the truth but remain unable to resist their urge to protect and provide.

Ed, described in Chapter 3, was the antisocial son of an influential judge whose money and connections likely contributed to his son's rambling course through life. The judge convinced his colleagues to ignore his son's minor criminal infractions, packed the boy off to a military academy, and later supported him through college and law school, all in the hope that Ed would straighten out under the right circumstances. He never did. Given the opportunity, an antisocial will take and take as long as he can, usually without any feeling of gratitude or indebtedness—at least none that lasts. Beginning in childhood, they become expert manipulators, developing skills that will be used throughout life to help them get what they want, honing them on well-meaning family members. Those born into wealth may keep drawing on family resources, able to avoid the demands of work and daily responsibilities that are major hurdles for most antisocials. Most such men never pause to consider how their comfortable family status carries them along, but if they did, they would probably just think themselves lucky. From a psychiatrist's perspective, however, the antisocial with an inherited safety net is actually unfortunate, because he is more likely to avoid the troublesome wake-up calls that spur others to make efforts to improve.

Compounding family loyalty and love is a desire to avoid the embarrassment that an antisocial family member can bring. For parents who have worked to attain success and respect, an antisocial son may be a burden worth hiding at almost any price, lest he reflect on their parenting skills and draw the scrutiny of friends and neighbors. Guilt helps keep ASP a secret since many parents of antisocial children, whether rich or poor, cannot help but think themselves somehow responsible for their child's problems. This mix of guilt, protective instincts, and the mistaken notion that criminal acts and antisocial behaviors occur only in poor or broken families conspires to maintain dangerous secrets. As long as antisocial behavior is regarded as a by-product of bad upbringing, social and economic deprivation, and other environmental factors, families are more likely to help middle- and upper-class antisocials hide from the world and from themselves.

Although efforts to protect a loved one are obviously not confined to any particular demographic group, not all families have the resources necessary to make them succeed. Take Alex Kelly for example. A young man from a wealthy Connecticut suburb who escaped rape charges for eight years by fleeing to Europe, Kelly provides an example of how well-to-do families can shelter members who engage in antisocial behavior.[3] Despite a past that included an alleged cocaine addiction funded by the theft of a reported $100,000 in property from neighborhood homes, the good-looking and ambitious Kelly remained a popular and successful son of his community, "a model student-athlete," according to a classmate quoted in a *Vanity Fair* article. He was a fierce competitor in his chosen sport of wrestling and an honor student with an A-minus average. But when he was accused of two brutal rapes within a week of each other, Kelly managed to disappear, with the knowledge and support of his parents, traveling abroad on money provided by them.

In 1995, he returned to stand trial and was convicted on one count of rape in a second trial after the first deadlocked. In the wake of the first trial, allegations of yet another rape surfaced, and Kelly was rearrested in his exclusive community on unrelated charges of disturbing the peace and leaving the scene of an accident. He pleaded not guilty to the charges. Kelly claimed that he had initially fled the country after his lawyer advised that being tried on two rape accusations before one jury—and before the media and community—was unfair. His years on the run over, Kelly still accepted little responsibility for his behavior. "I wasn't trying to get away from anything," he said in a televised interview. "Why should I go to jail for something I didn't do?"[4]

The Kelly case brought a flood of media attention, some of it seeming to revel in the purported exposure of a wealthy community striving to maintain cherished illusions of privacy and respectability. Kelly's parents—if not the young man himself—were supported by some neighbors who professed to understand their dilemma. What, they asked themselves, would they have done were it their son? Like the William Kennedy Smith rape trial years before, Kelly's story was irresistible to reporters, who saw it as an opportunity to dig into the dark side of a prosperous family. This relentless interest in scandal may provide a further incentive for those families of antisocials who have the means to keep secrets and avoid public humiliation. If stories of drug use, burglary, and rape from Kelly's past are to be believed, his flight from prosecution reflects a recurrent effort to keep his troubles quiet and maintain the semblance of normality. However, although some may sympathize with the Kellys, protecting a family member with a tendency toward antisocial behavior may have destructive consequences.

Hidden behind walls insulated with money, fear, and guilt, antisocial behavior can build in a family to the point of explosion, sometimes culminating in tragedy. When violence erupts from homes of wealth and power, it tends to make headlines. One of the most notorious examples—as well as the one with the most relevance to ASP—is that of Lyle and Erik Menendez, convicted of the 1989 shotgun murders of their parents in the family's Beverly Hills mansion.

It was perfect fodder for sensationalized media coverage, but the scene of the crime and the substantial inheritance that fell into the brothers' hands drew much greater attention to the case than to similar offenses committed under different circumstances. In 1997, two teenage brothers in New Hampshire received prison terms for killing their parents.[5] According to court testimony, the elder brother had claimed that he wanted to shoot their mother to see the look on her face, to which the younger replied, "Why do you get all the fun?" After the killings, the boys hid the bodies and spent a weekend partying with friends before returning to school the following Monday. Although reported nationally, the case got much less news coverage than the Menendez trial, perhaps because there was little money involved. Initially disregarded as suspects in the case, the Menendez brothers had raised suspicions by spending $700,000 of their inheritance in the weeks after the killings and had confessed under police questioning.[6] Prosecutors maintained that greed drove the brothers to murder their parents for the $14 million family fortune. The brothers' attorneys countered that the slayings were committed in self-defense after years of physical and sexual abuse, although their clients had made no effort to escape the allegedly abusive environment, even as young men. The original jury was unable to reach a verdict, but a second trial ended in conviction after the judge excluded many of the abuse claims. The two were sentenced to life in prison with no chance of parole.

Like the story of Alex Kelly, the Menendez case illustrates how antisocial behavior draws extra attention when it occurs high on the socioeconomic ladder. It is also another instance in which ASP—rather than childhood abuse—may be the key to understanding how such a crime could happen. Both Lyle and Erik Menendez had a history of trouble. As teenagers, they were involved in a series of burglaries that netted more than $100,000 from the houses of their friends' parents. Lyle was involved in another burglary after going away to college at Princeton, where he was suspended during his freshman year for cheating. During their first murder trial, Erik's high-profile attorney, Leslie Abramson, had a description of the brothers as "sociopaths" ruled inadmissible. Although I cannot say whether the Menendez brothers are antisocial, their histories show clues that would be notable in any psychiatric assessment. Certainly, the brothers' actions related to the crime—the bloody killings, a feigned 911 call, the reckless spending of newly acquired wealth—fit a pattern of misbehavior that is conspicuously antisocial.

Although this story might have received less attention had Lyle and Erik Menendez come from another background—or been less photogenic—it is also possible that the murders might never have occurred under different circumstances. Whatever preceded the crime—be it years of abuse, greed, antisocial behavior, or something altogether different—money and status may have shielded it from view. Perhaps, in another family of less means, the problem might have come to light before it was too late.

SUCCESSFUL BAD BOYS

Antisocials are not just muggers, rapists, and violent assailants. They sometimes are embezzlers, tax evaders, fraudulent business-men, corrupt stock brokers, and conniving attorneys. Antisocials who habitually commit white-collar crimes may be more likely to escape prosecution or punishment, especially if they also manage to maintain an aura of success and influential connections. Those who evade capture or conduct their professional lives with a modicum of integrity may not show the most obvious, public symptoms of ASP. Their nature may be expressed more destructively in other behaviors, including domestic abuse, neglect of children, drug use, or even a habit of reckless driving.

Most antisocials, however, have little luck with conventional occupations and career demands, so those who manage to find suc-cess may do so by alternate routes, some of them illegal. The success-ful con man or white-collar criminal may seem like a run-of-the-mill husband and father to his neighbors, so long as they refrain from asking too many questions about what he does for a living or how he manages to afford an unusually expensive lifestyle. An example of such a man was recently profiled on the television program *American Greed*. Raffaello Follieri, a 29-year-old entrepreneur, seemed to have it all—movie star looks, a successful real business, and an A-list girl-friend, the actress Anne Hathaway.[7] While hobnobbing with the wealthy and connected, his business empire came crashing down when he was revealed to be a con man who was racking up huge debts to sustain a lifestyle that included whisking his girlfriend around the world on chartered jets, staying at the Dorchester Hotel in London, and living in a duplex apartment that overlooked New York's St. Patrick's Cathedral. From humble beginnings, the hot-tempered Italian sought to make his mark on the world. He concocted a scheme to mislead investors and convince them of his special relationship with the Vatican, one that allowed him to buy church property at discounted prices. Dubbed the "Vati-con" by the tabloids, Follieri went so far as to claim that he met with the Pope whenever he was in Rome. Arrested on charges of wire fraud and money laundering, and having been abandoned by his actress girlfriend, Follieri eventually pleaded guilty and was sentenced to four-and-a-half years in prison.

Another noteworthy con man, Richard Bailey, was convicted of conspiring to murder candy heiress Helen Vorhees Brach, who van-ished in 1977.[8] A former vacuum cleaner salesman and TV repairman, Bailey pleaded guilty to federal racketeering charges and admitted defrauding more than a dozen women but maintained his innocence in connection with the Brach case. His favorite targets were wealthy widows or divorcees whom he met at bars, restaurants, horse shows, or through personal ads. After showering them with charm, vows of love, and sometimes marriage proposals, he persuaded them to invest in overvalued horses like the nine he sold Helen Brach before she dis-appeared. Bailey's other schemes included driving schools, smoking clinics, a fast food restaurant, and a depilatory cream that he adver-tised with vanity plates reading "SHAVE IT" on his red Mercedes. "I'm a good salesman, if that's what they call a con man," Bailey told one writer who investigated the Brach disappearance. "If I was a con man, I'd never have been involved in all these businesses."

Maybe it is the appeal of getting something for nothing or a grudging respect for the ability to sweet talk one's way to prosperity, but antisocial con artists are sometimes seen as harmless, if not likable, rogues. Some observers understand or even admire their brazen actions, especially when they involve avoiding taxes, defrauding big business, or otherwise taking money from a faceless government or corporation. These and other forms of antisocial behavior somehow strike a chord with various facets of the public imagination, whether it is the blend of fascination and dread roused by lurid accounts of murder or the adolescent envy of individuals who perpetually flout the rules and get away with it. For some, public displays of antisocial behavior can, in fact, be quite profitable.

Perhaps each of us is a little bit antisocial. We are born into a world of norms and regulations that most of us internalize, but which doesn't make us immune to the urge to sometimes break the rules or get away with something a bit shady. For most people, violations are relatively minor and infrequent—an unpaid parking ticket here, unreported income there—and most customs and laws are understood to serve a purpose and promote social stability. Although individuals interpret and respond to rules in different ways, most of us are guided by a conscience that is perhaps both biologically and socially determined, enabling us to live within legal, religious, and ethical boundaries. Although the antisocial who lacks a moral compass to guide his behavior may remind us of the value of social regulation, to some extent he is also a reminder of the appeal that flouting the law has at times to even the most normal of us.

Antisocial behavior is valued to a degree in certain contexts, and a few professions offer opportunities for antisocials to succeed by expressing tendencies that would be discouraged elsewhere. Despite its rigid discipline and strict regulations, military service offers some antisocials a chance to put their violent streak to work, as in the case of "Dirty Jim," profiled in Chapter 5. Similarly, whether it's on the field, rink, or ring, competitive sports reward behavior that would otherwise be considered antisocial. Although both professions accept and even reward antisocial behavior so long as it stays in check, they police themselves for instances when such behavior crosses established lines. Peacetime acts of violence among members of the military provoke outrage and swift punishment. Crimes committed by athletes can bring professional sanctions or civil penalties when they violate codes of conduct. Witness pro basketball player Latrell Sprewell's suspension for attacking his coach, or boxer Mike Tyson's sanction for biting off part of an opponent's ear.[9] Even the most aggressive sports set up rules that some individuals have trouble obeying.

In sports, music, movies, and other forms of entertainment, a clear market for professional bad boys exists, and plenty of candidates are eager to fill the demand. Are these men simply shrewd operators cashing in on society's perpetual interest in bad behavior, or are they true antisocials who have somehow managed to find their niche? In 1996, recording artist Tupac Shakur was shot to death in Las Vegas.[10] A star in the world of gangsta rap, a musical style born of inner-city violence and deprivation, Shakur died a death not unlike those described in his music. His mother was a member of the Black Panther party, acquitted on bombing and conspiracy charges while carrying Shakur, whose father she could not identify. Born in New York, Shakur was introduced to life on the streets of Harlem and later attended the prestigious High School for the Performing Arts in Baltimore. After moving to Marin City, California, with his mother and sister, Shakur attended an upscale high school before dropping out and entering the drug trade. Soon, however, he began his rise as a rapper and actor, and his troubles seemed to deepen even as his career developed. He was incarcerated briefly in 1994, after a fist fight with a film director, and later that year returned to jail on a sexual abuse conviction. Also in 1994, he was seriously wounded in a shooting ambush. His music and lifestyle may have provoked the assault, as his recordings and public statements were peppered with insults and intimidation aimed at rivals.

Some might argue that Shakur's misbehavior stemmed from a difficult childhood and the machismo-fueled fashion of gangsta rap, noting that his descent into "thug life"—the motto tattooed across his abdomen—accompanied his success. Regardless of the causes behind his actions, Shakur's stardom demonstrates that antisocial behavior can sell records and help construct a marketable public persona. With a little talent or sheer luck, an antisocial just might find a career in which the darker elements of his personality cease to matter. Although I suspect that truly antisocial athletes and performers are rare, I believe that they and those who act like them have found a place in the media-saturated culture of celebrity. They are afforded the latitude to act out in exchange for symbolizing what some of their fans may crave but can never have—freedom to live beyond the rules. Critics maintain that this glorification of antisocial behavior in the world of entertainment spawns real-world imitators, particularly among the young. Indeed, professional bad boys find a ready-made audience in young people, especially males, some of whom are primed for rebellion in any package.

THE PROBLEM OF ADULT ANTISOCIAL BEHAVIOR

When I read about Bernie Madoff's pyramid scheme, which bilked thousands of investors of hard earned savings to the tune of $65 billion, or people like Raffaello Follieri, whose wild schemes have ended the dreams of many, I wonder if the person has ASP written all through his personal history. Was he a bad boy who grew up to be a bad man? Was he a good man gone wrong? If so, how and why did he change from the presumably good person he was? If there is no history of prior behavioral problems, whether in his personal life or among his business ventures, could this be a form of ASP?

The psychiatric field has struggled to answer these questions, and the American Psychiatric Association's *Diagnostic and Statistical Manual of Mental Disorders, Fourth Edition, Text Revision (DSM-IV-TR)* considers such scenarios evidence of *adult antisocial behavior,* a category "used when the focus of clinical attention is ... not due to a mental disorder."[11] Thus, from the *DSM* standpoint, adult antisocial behavior does not rise to the level of a mental disorder, even though it may be troublesome to the individual and the community. Professional thieves, racketeers, or dealers in illegal substances—in other words, the Bernie Madoffs of the world—are examples of persons who might merit this designation. What separates these people from the true antisocial is the lack of a background of early misconduct. Without the history of longstanding behavioral problems dating to childhood or early adolescence, the presumption is that these are fundamentally normal people gone wrong.

Bernie Madoff, a former chairman of NASDAQ, is the perfect example because there is no evidence I've seen that he was troubled as a youth.[12] Instead, Madoff had an unremarkable childhood as one of three children in a modest Queens, New York family, went to Hofstra, and scrimped and saved as a lifeguard in Far Rockaway. After graduating in 1960, Madoff founded an investment firm that eventually became his downfall after it was discovered that he had systematically defrauded thousands of investors—including some of his closest friends—in one of the largest Ponzi schemes in the history of finance. The firm was a family affair, and offered trades and markets in securities that outpaced his competition, attracting investors from among the wealthy and powerful Madoff knew on the Upper East

Side, the Hamptons, Palm Beach, or the south of France. In 2009, he pleaded guilty to 11 federal felonies and was sentenced to 150 years in prison. The great mystery to those following the case was his elusive personality. Asked about the deviant workings of the singular criminal mind, psychologist Stanton E. Samenow, quoted in *Vanity Fair*, describes many as appearing outwardly normal, but "their self-esteem rises or falls at the expense of another. Bernie Madoff shares personality traits with embezzlers and serial killers."

Risë Goldstein, a researcher with the National Institute of Alcohol Abuse and Alcoholism, who has studied this issue, concludes that there is a full spectrum of antisocial behavior in the general population, with adult antisocial behavior at the less severe end. Whether adult antisocial behavior will ever be considered a clinical disorder remains uncertain, although it clearly describes many people and causes much grief.[13]

AN ANTISOCIAL IN HIDING

Cathy parked her car along the curb, an expansive stretch of close-cropped lawn between her and the home of Richard White, who had been admitted to the University of Iowa's psychiatric ward more than 20 years earlier after drinking a bottle of rubbing alcohol. The house was low and wide, like many in the neighborhood, trimmed with carefully groomed foliage. A Volvo station wagon and a BMW sedan rested in the driveway. The only sounds were the laughter of a child from a distant backyard and the purring of a neighbor's lawn mower.

Richard greeted her at the door. He was 42 years old, but slim and athletic. He was dressed in a dark suit, pressed white shirt, and red silk tie, clothes that prompted Cathy to suspect he was either a businessman or a funeral director. Although we had little trouble finding him through credit bureau records, we had no idea how he made his living. His home and cars hinted that whatever he did rewarded him well. He welcomed her into a stylish and comfortable living room and politely asked her the first question: Why would she possibly care to interview him? Cathy offered him a printed summary of the study, titled "Life Adjustment of Formerly Hospitalized Patients," and a consent form. He glanced over both and signed the form with a fountain pen produced from his jacket pocket, then sat back in his chair, crossed his legs, and invited her to begin.

Cathy asked whether he recalled being in the hospital in 1966. He paused as if searching for a distant memory, then began to answer slowly, perhaps afraid of revealing too much too fast. He remembered, he said, but felt the need to explain. The incident had been a cry for help, not a suicide attempt, and he had thought that downing the rubbing alcohol would communicate his distress. His records showed that the event had been brought on by his second wife's request for a divorce, and the admitting physician wrote that Richard had a 10- to 15-year history of "fighting and aggressive behavior, emotional instability, and antisocial acts. ... He has been married for the second time and has committed adultery leading to upheaval and tension in the marriage. He has had many jobs and has been fired from a few."

Richard's memory of the hospital stay conflicted with the record. While he claimed to have been there two weeks, he was actually released after five days. The physicians found him well-mannered, friendly, and cooperative, with no sign of delusions, hallucinations, or phobias, or any ongoing depression or suicidal thinking. In fact, he seemed to identify his own problem, describing "his poor behavior throughout his life and his desire to obtain psychiatric help in making better decisions in the future." There was no apparent medical explanation for his actions, and although the doctors deferred in making a diagnosis, they noted that his long history of "acting out behavior, impulsivity, emotional immaturity, and poor judgment would lead one to suspect a sociopathic personality disturbance." Richard's wife had no patience for their jargon, insisting that there was nothing wrong with her husband aside from a need to grow up and accept responsibility. Having reconciled for the moment, the couple left the hospital together.

Digging deeper, Cathy asked about his childhood. Richard claimed to have a poor memory—contrary to hospital records citing his excellent recall—and insisted that he had deliberately blocked out much of his past with an abusive alcoholic father and an equally unpredictable mother. As a child, he had been troubled by nightmares and constant fights between his parents, who sometimes lashed out at him for offenses as mild as forgetting to wash his hands. Ashamed of his father, who swung from meek to belligerent depending on his degree of drunkenness, and frightened of his oppressive mother, Richard learned to lurk quietly around the home, avoiding both of them as much as possible. At school, however, he mouthed off to teachers, fought with other boys, and neglected his work, blaming someone else for each of his problems. Persistent truancy forced him to repeat 9th grade, and he dropped out when told he would have to do 10th grade over as well.

When 14, his mother's temper cooled after she claimed to have had a vision of Jesus Christ. At about the same time, Richard's father stopped drinking, but Richard's own misbehavior continued. He admitted to Cathy that he had joined a gang after leaving school but maintained that he had no trouble with the law until age 19. The psychiatric records showed a more complete version of his youthful misadventures. They include his descriptions of "messing around with girls" and picking up gay men in order to rob them, a habit that led to an assault and battery arrest after he savagely beat a man outside a bar. The charges were dropped when he enlisted in the Marines, but he received a medical discharge after only five months of service.

According to his records, Richard eventually married three times, the first to a woman he had known for only three weeks. Although only 18, she had been married three times before meeting Richard, and their relationship dissolved after nine months of mistrust and infidelity. During that period, Richard managed to move through four or five jobs, complaining that he hated either the work or his co-workers. Two of his wife's brothers joined him in a burglary spree that ended in arrest and a short jail term, and his wife was gone by the time he was released. He quickly remarried but remained sexually unsatisfied, cruising local bars for willing young women and eventually disappearing for days at a time without explanation.

His life changed, he told Cathy, when he was "born again" at age 28. He took up serious Bible study and was ordained as a Pentecostal minister. The religious experience led him to view his past behavior in a new light. Where he had once blamed parents, teachers, and any other available scapegoat, he now blamed—or rather credited—God for the choices he had made. When Cathy asked about his sexual history, Richard steadfastly explained that he was "God's vessel" and had a duty to provide his seed to women. He was proud to have fathered four children within his marriages and several out of wedlock, although the only two with whom he had contact had come out of his current marriage. Although he claimed to feel bad about abandoning his other children, he saw no need to provide them with financial support. After all, he had done his deed by siring them.

His years of alcohol and drug addiction were also part of God's plan. Richard recalled once being drunk "for an entire year" and volunteered that he had sold drugs for a period, falling into a habit that had "nearly destroyed" his life. Although he swore that he had given it all up, he still feared that the authorities were looking for him. He had developed peptic ulcers and clinical depression, but said that God had healed him and would speak to him in times of need.

Since leaving the Marines in his late teens, Richard had held 40 to 50 jobs—pumping gas, waiting tables, detassling corn, working in construction—many lasting only days. He recalled at least 15 in the decade before the interview, causing Cathy to wonder how he had managed to acquire his home and cars, considering such an unstable work history. In addition to his part-time pastoral work, he claimed to be employed as a barber, although he did not explain where or when he had received his training. Besides, Cathy thought, how many barbers drive BMWs? Was he still dealing drugs or engaged in some other illegal activity? Had he married into money?

Unfortunately, her final questions were never asked or answered. Richard cut the interview short, suddenly announcing that his wife would be home soon and that Cathy would have to leave. She gathered her things, wondering if she had come too close to discovering a truth that he preferred to keep hidden. Although Richard had claimed to have no secrets from his wife, he seemed concerned that she might discover an unknown aspect of his checkered past. As he showed Cathy to the door, Richard brushed a hand against her arm and asked why she had conducted the interview alone: "How did you know you would be safe and I wouldn't pull something on you?" Cathy declined to answer, instead thanking him for his time and rushing to her car, waiting for the sound of his door shutting behind her. She saw him watching from the window, then drawing the blinds as she pulled into the quiet street.

Richard had all the trappings of a comfortable middle-class existence, but his sly evasions, transparent half-truths, and plain lack of remorse indicated that he had not changed. Although he did not come from money, had never finished high school, and offered no evidence of career success, he had somehow managed to attain a lifestyle that would be the envy of many. We were left to wonder whether he supported himself through crime or the generosity of a doting wife, and also whether he was able to sustain his apparent success.

Chapter 9

The Antisocial Murderer

Gacy and Others

THE DISCOVERY

They descended on the house, a 1950s brick ranch home in an unincorporated neighborhood outside Chicago. Police cars and dozens of officers swarmed over the property, drawing the attention of puzzled neighbors and soon the media. Inside, pictures of clowns hung from the walls, along with photographs showing the home's owner, a pudgy contractor named John Gacy, with the mayor of Chicago and Rosalynn Carter, wife of President Jimmy Carter.[1] Investigators searched the house and garage, finding wallets and jewelry that had belonged to several teenage boys, but the focus of attention was a crawl space below the front of the house. There, masked men huddled beneath the floorboards and footfalls, examining a carefully sketched map and slowly scraping away the putrid muck, as if on an archaeological dig. The house was built above a reclaimed marsh, and fetid puddles of water swimming with worms splashed under their hands and feet. Soon they began bringing up the bodies. Some were little more than skeletons, their flesh dissolved into a foamy white substance. The stench forced police to dig in shifts, taking frequent breaks to come up for air and a brief respite from the grim discovery. Eventually, they pulled 25 corpses from the crawl space and recovered another four from elsewhere on the property. In a matter of hours, an ordinary, middle-class home had become known as the site of unspeakable horror.

It was late December 1978, and news from the scene reached a nation occupied with holiday plans and thoughts of a new year. Police in Des Plaines, Illinois, had zeroed in on Gacy while probing the disappearance of a 15-year-old boy last seen leaving to speak with him about a job. With his history of arrests for crimes involving young men, Gacy soon became a suspect in the case and the subject of round-the-clock surveillance, despite his vehement denials of any wrongdoing. Days later, a search warrant produced evidence of bodies buried in Gacy's crawl space and, under interrogation, the contractor admitted to luring more than 30 young men and boys to his home with promises of high-paying construction work. There he would handcuff, rape, and torture them, finally ending their brutal ordeal by knotting a rope around their necks and twisting it tight with a hammer handle or by cramming their underwear deep into their throats until they suffocated.[2] He then buried the bodies in shallow trenches below the house, sprinkling them with lime or acid to speed decomposition. When the crawl space grew crowded with graves, Gacy dumped his last four victims in the Des Plaines River. On two or three occasions, he murdered two men in one night—"doubles" as he called them.

At the time of his arrest and conviction, Gacy was the most prolific serial killer in American history, and he remains one of the best-known members of a hideous fraternity—men who kill again and again, often for no apparent motive. Despite differences, their biographies often read like textbook studies of antisocial personality disorder (ASP) manifested in a most deadly way. Not all serial killers are antisocial and, certainly, few antisocials rise to the heights of violence reached by men like Gacy, Jeffrey Dahmer, Ted Bundy, Henry Lee Lucas, and David Berkowitz. But ASP symptoms—unruly childhoods, failures at school and work, legal skirmishes, instability, impulsiveness, and the like—are common themes in their lives.

In 1968, only a few years before the killings began and following a sodomy charge, Gacy had been diagnosed as antisocial at the University of Iowa, so he was a perfect candidate for my study. Gacy lore had circulated around the institution since his murder arrest, and I was eager to search his records for any sign that might have foretold his violent turn. I was even more intrigued by the prospect of interviewing him. Finding the infamous murderer was easy; he was a death row inmate at the Menard Correctional Center in Springfield, Illinois. In early 1987, Sue attempted to arrange an interview, first writing to the center's director about the possibility of a meeting. "I do not feel it [would] be productive for the Department of Corrections or Mr. Gacy to have any special attention directed towards him," the director wrote, prompting us to contact Gacy's attorney and then to write to the killer directly. One week after sending him a letter outlining the study and the importance of his participation, we received this reply:

> My attorneys inform me while my appeal is pending that I cannot assist in your study since you're in my transcripts as not being reliable, and that your doctors are paid professional witnesses.

We let the matter rest, writing again eight months later. By that time, his appeal to the United States Supreme Court had been rejected. Perhaps Gacy would now feel free to participate. Two weeks later, on June 8, 1989, we received his response:

> Sorry to disappoint you.... I have enclosed a copy of the typical route of a capital case on appeal. The news media just likes to see my name in print, or they are hard up for news. In any case my appeal just finished step number four, so you can read on from there.
>
> Regarding any interviews, those requests go through my attorney or agent in New York, the fee is $500 a minute for the first hour which has to be paid in advance for the first hour, and the money goes to charity. It is the same kind of fees doctors are paid for being professional witnesses, and just as unreliable as to what will be said, according to whose side they are on.
>
> Have a nice day.

He signed the letter with a flourish and indicated that a carbon copy would be placed in a file labeled PEOPLE UP TO NO GOOD. A complicated algorithm for appealing capital cases in seven separate steps accompanied the letter. It was our last contact with Gacy.

Gacy's notoriety made it easy to assess his life after psychiatric hospitalization, even without his assistance. As one of the most highly profiled killers in the annals of American crime, he was the focus of books, magazine stories, newspaper articles, and even an eerie following. According to a 1988 news story, Gacy received nearly a dozen letters each day, many of them interested in his paintings of clowns and other subjects.[3] More than 400 of his works were sold— even more after his eventual execution—and he was once invited by a religious group to design Christmas cards. He also found time for a jailhouse romance with a woman from Centralia, Illinois, to whom he proposed marriage. She described Gacy as "real soft spoken, real kind," dismissing the evidence against him: "From what I've read and everything, it wasn't investigated very good.... To me he don't seem like he could hurt anyone." Despite his initial confession, Gacy denied committing his crimes until the end, spouting theories of what could have happened, making unconvincing attempts to feign mental illness, and even proclaiming his innocence on a 900 telephone line that charged callers $1.99 per minute.[4]

Gacy's crimes brought him a sordid sort of fame, as his name became synonymous with the term *serial killer*. His years spent languishing on death row protesting his conviction and constantly promoting himself make Gacy an enduring symbol even after his death. To many, Gacy represents the worst kind of criminal, a man who methodically carried out torture and killings but never admitted a shred of remorse, instead taunting society and the families of his victims for as long as he could. Although found guilty on the basis of his own confession and the discovery of some 29 bodies on his property, Gacy claimed he was the true victim and continued to evade responsibility, as he had his entire life. Yet, Gacy sometimes showed remarkable ambition and even generosity, although his small successes were built on a precarious foundation of moral apathy and pathological self-absorption. He was convinced that he could take whatever he wanted, even when that meant taking lives.

WATERLOO

A decade before his arrest for murder, Gacy, then 26, had made a name for himself in Waterloo, Iowa, a working-class town, where he managed a string of Kentucky Fried Chicken restaurants owned by his father-in-law. In the two years since his arrival in town, Gacy had become chaplain of the local Junior Chamber of Commerce and organizer of the group's first communitywide prayer breakfast. He hosted backyard barbecues for his widening circle of friends, sent buckets of chicken to the local boys' club, and volunteered to shop for Christmas presents for underprivileged children. He also joined the Merchant's Patrol, a loosely knit but officially sanctioned volunteer group organized to help police area businesses. A hard worker and tireless community organizer, Gacy earned the respect of his neighbors and colleagues, living comfortably with his wife and two children in a bungalow on the city's west side. Even critics of his shameless self-promotion and swaggering manner had to admit that when there was a job to be done, Gacy was the man to call.

But Gacy's outward success shielded secret passions that were exposed once he was accused of molesting a teenage boy. The incident became the talk of Waterloo, splitting supporters, who noted Gacy's record of community service, from detractors outraged by the allegations. The latter complained that Gacy had always acted with a roguish bluster and told outright lies, including claims that the governor of Illinois had appointed him to several important committees. Authorities alleged that Gacy had used such lies to coerce the 16-year-old son of a fellow Jaycee into repeated acts of oral sex. The boy's story was bolstered by that of another youth, one of Gacy's employees, who revealed that his boss had made sexual propositions and threatened him with a knife when he declined. Before long, both boys were sharing their stories with parents and police, leading to a grand jury investigation. Gacy swore his innocence and demanded a polygraph test, eventually undergoing two and failing both. Locals soon joked that the only answer Gacy got right was his name.

Gacy brought further trouble upon himself during the investigation. He invited a young employee, a high school football player, to accompany him on his Merchant Patrol rounds. After breaking into a lumber store and burglarizing an auto dealer—perhaps to seal a bond between them—Gacy offered the athlete $300 to beat up the boy who had leveled the molestation charge, hoping to stop him from testifying. The beating took place the next day and was promptly reported to the police, who questioned the assailant until he identified Gacy as the instigator. Facing additional charges of going armed with intent, making malicious threats to extort, and attempting to suborn perjury—as well as breaking and entering from the lumber store incident—Gacy was jailed, unable to raise bail.

In a clumsy attempt to defend himself, Gacy spun a convoluted tale of conspiracy and political intrigue, claiming his accuser's father was a rival Jaycee who had set him up in order to further his own ambitions. A police raid on Gacy's home that produced "planted" pornographic films was part of the story. Gacy also denied involvement in the breaking and entering incident and the ensuing assault. When pressed, he reluctantly admitted to having oral sex with his accuser on a few occasions, motivated, he claimed, by innocent curiosity. He changed his story several times to paint the boy as the one who had initiated the sex in exchange for various sums of money. The relationship surfaced, Gacy claimed, after a failed extortion attempt. In Gacy's account, someone else was always to blame.

In reality, the charges against him only hinted at Gacy's illicit activities. He organized not only barbecues and prayer breakfasts, but also a clandestine "social club" for local youths, a trap for any who would submit to his sexual advances. Boys who paid small monthly dues were welcomed to a basement rec room stocked with beer and liquor and equipped with a pool table and projector for screening pornographic films. Gacy boasted about so-called sex research commissioned by the governor of Illinois and challenged boys to games of pool in exchange for oral sex. Those who refused were promised the services of his wife, whereas others who rebuffed all such advances were warned that unspecified people from Chicago would get rid of them if they informed. Some actually believed Gacy's con and had sex with him, but few ever came forward to admit it.

Based on testimony from the boys who had told, Gacy was indicted and ordered by a judge to undergo psychiatric assessment at the University of Iowa Psychopathic Hospital. Upon arrival, he was taken to one of two locked inpatient units, where he immediately began ingratiating himself with the nursing staff. He boasted to the other patients of the money he made and the cars he owned, and insisted that he was a victim, not a criminal. Used to taking charge, Gacy set out to prove himself helpful to the ward staff and, by the second week, was calling himself the "barn boss."[5] As told in *Buried Dreams*, Gacy asserted authority over the other patients: "Sometimes, yes, he had to bark at them, but only as a last recourse.... Sometimes he felt as if he was 'running the whole place by myself.'" He even manipulated one fellow patient into making his bed.[6]

BIRTH OF A KILLER

Gacy's busy efforts to occupy his time and impress the hospital staff in the same way he had the people of Waterloo were wasted on his doctors. They conducted tests, performed examinations, and initiated interviews that revealed pieces of Gacy's life, beginning with his youth in Chicago. The son of strict Polish-Catholic immigrants, Gacy's father was a harsh disciplinarian and an abusive drunk who hid his brandy in the basement and was quick to apply his razor strop to a child caught misbehaving. He once knocked out several of his wife's teeth during a fight and beat or bullied his son John for various offenses—whether or not the boy was responsible. Terrified of his father's unpredictable violence, Gacy grew up close to his mother and two sisters, only to be called a mama's boy or a sissy by his father. He sought refuge at the Catholic schools he attended until age 11 and developed a reputation as friendly, easygoing, and bright. But when the family moved and he entered public school, John seemed to lose interest, skipping classes and ignoring his studies.

He grew up with chronic health problems that were never fully explained and were an additional source of friction with his father, who insisted that John faked his symptoms to get out of school. Born a "blue baby"—which usually indicates a congenital defect of the heart—John was ordered by doctors not to play sports or engage in strenuous physical activity, thus setting him apart from his peers. By age 10, he was having fainting spells for no apparent reason, sometimes accompanied by rapid breathing. Between the ages of 18 and 20, he was hospitalized for more than 200 days and told that he suffered from "psychomotor epilepsy due to hyperventilation" whenever he got excited. Similar problems continued for years, leading to later hospitalizations for attacks of "nerves" or "mild strokes."[7] His expanding bulk also underscored his difference from the other boys. By age 18, his 5-foot, 8-inch frame ballooned to 200 pounds.

At age 14, John was transferred to a vocational school, probably due to his record of truancy and indifferent grades. He became a favorite of his teachers and performed better in this less competitive environment, ranking first in his class of 79 students. A civil defense captain at his school and the founder of a young adults' club at church, John considered joining the priesthood. But, for unexplained reasons, he changed schools an additional three times and eventually dropped out altogether. He had other troubles as well, later admitting to lying and stealing that began at age six—when he took a toy truck from a discount store—and continued into his teens and adulthood.

The strained relationship with his father drove Gacy to leave home—"running away," he called it, even though he was 20 years old at the time. He landed in Las Vegas, where he briefly found work as a mortuary attendant, sleeping on a cot behind the embalming room. In *Buried Dreams*, Gacy is said to have recounted erotic attractions to the corpses of young men, which he found even more troublesome than the terrifying feelings he once had for male friends, but none of this emerged during his 1968 assessment.[8] Instead, Gacy traced his path back to Illinois and minor success. Realizing that his life was going nowhere, Gacy had managed to save enough money to return home and enroll at Northwestern Business College for a one-year course. After graduating with good grades, he secured a job as a management trainee with Nunn-Bush shoes and was transferred to Springfield, Illinois, which became the opportunity he had sought. He refined his talent for manipulation through his dealings with customers, later boasting to have increased shoe sales by 40%, and he married the daughter of a local businessman.

Within a month of his wedding, Gacy had his first sexual experience with a man, a friend who offered oral sex when the two of them were drunk.[9] Gacy claimed to have disliked the experience, insisting that his later sexual relations with men stemmed from curiosity rather than repressed homosexual impulses. He hated gay men, he told his doctors, especially effeminate or flamboyant ones. He first had sex with a woman at age 18 and had been sexually involved with several others before marrying at age 24. With women, he preferred "normal sex" to oral intercourse, as the latter left him unable to kiss his female partners afterward. He would later explain his pursuit of male sex partners as a way of finding physical gratification without emotional involvement—little more than masturbation, as he saw it. Asked about the sodomy charge and how it fit into his pattern of desire, Gacy tried to portray his behavior as routine in a freewheeling community of businessmen who regularly consorted with prostitutes and slept with each other's wives. None of the other Jaycees, however, were being arrested for molesting boys.

DIAGNOSIS

A battery of medical tests—including an electroencephalogram (EEG), skull x-rays, and blood draws to rule out syphilis and diabetes—failed to reveal any disease or disability and, aside from his obesity, Gacy was deemed physically normal.[10] He remained "relaxed and reasonably sincere" during the mental status examination, and his doctors summarized their findings: "His affect is appropriate without evidence of depression, anxiety, or suspicion. His associations are intact, however, his answers tend to be rather circular." Gacy's IQ score was 118, placing him in the "bright normal range," and his highest verbal test score was in comprehension, "indicating a high degree of social intelligence or awareness of the proper way to behave to influence others."

But Gacy had not fooled staff psychologist Eugene R. Gauron. "It was apparent that John would twist the truth in such a way that he would not be made to look bad," Gauron wrote. He continued with an assessment that would prove a disturbingly apt description of Gacy's destructive personality:

> The most shocking aspect of the test results is the patient's total denial of responsibility for anything that has happened to him. He can produce an alibi for everything. He alternatively blames the environment while presenting himself as a victim of circumstances and blames other people while presenting himself as the victim of others who are out to get him.... A second feature of the test results is the patient's propensity to behave impulsively. He often does things without thinking through the consequences and exercises poor judgment in the bargain.

Test results indicated antisocial personality, Gauron concluded, but not "unusual thought processes." In other words, Gacy was responsible for his behavior and knew what he was doing. He simply refused to admit it.

Staff psychiatrist Leonard Heston and resident Larry Amick agreed with the diagnosis, defining ASP as a "term reserved for individuals who are basically unsocialized and whose behavior pattern brings them repeatedly into conflict with society. Persons with this personality structure do not learn from experience and are unlikely to benefit from known medical treatment." Amick later described Gacy as "completely untrustworthy," without any apparent "appreciation for what was socially acceptable and what was unacceptable." The doctors concluded that Gacy was mentally competent to stand trial. Writing to the judge who ordered the exam, they noted that similar antisocials "do best when there are firm, consistent external controls on their behavior." Gacy's stable work record was a good sign, they thought, adding that "it would give [him] a little better prognosis than most other persons of his personality type."

Gacy went on to plead guilty to the charges and put himself at the court's mercy. A presentence investigator recommended parole, noting Gacy's solid record of work and community service and his insistence that encounters with the boy were an "experiment." The judge saw things differently. On December 3, 1968, he sentenced a stunned Gacy to 10 years at the Iowa Men's Reformatory in Anamosa. Although acknowledging that incarceration may not be the best answer, the judge told Gacy that prison would "ensure for some period of time that you cannot seek out teenage boys to solicit them for immoral behavior of any kind."

Behind bars, Gacy became a model prisoner. He started a Jaycee chapter, resumed his old duties as chaplain, worked in the prison kitchen, organized Jaycee banquets, and played Santa Claus at Christmas, all while managing to finish his high school studies. His efforts brought him the Jaycee Sound Citizens Award and other honors while in jail, as well as an early release for good behavior after 16 months. Once paroled, he was allowed to return to Chicago to live with his mother. A year and a half later, John Gacy would kill the first of his 33 victims.

READING THE SIGNS

Although national interest in Gacy has faded now that it has been nearly 20 years since his execution, Gacy is still talked about at the University of Iowa—one of those notorious cases sometimes used to illustrate a particular disorder. But if Gacy had not gone on to become a serial murderer, his story would likely be lost among thousands of psychiatric records. If anything set him apart from his fellow antisocials, it was his professional ambition and ability to weave his way into a community, attributes not commonly found in men with ASP. In fact, Gacy was on his way to becoming a relatively high-functioning antisocial when his façade was shattered by the sodomy conviction. Gacy would attempt to pick up the pieces and begin a new life at home in Chicago, but it eventually became clear that this chapter marked a turn for the worse.

In 1968, Gacy's doctors assessed him in much the way that their counterparts would today, identifying their patient's ASP and recommending strong sanctions to hold him accountable for his behavior. They described what seemed to be mitigating factors in his disorder and expressed a guarded prognosis, acknowledging the possibility that he might improve. When I review their notes I am struck by the prescience of their observations, but cannot help wonder if there is something they might have missed and whether I may have overlooked something similar in one of my own patients. Antisocial personality disorder tends to follow a predictable pattern of misbehavior that may taper over time but usually remains the source of lifelong problems.

Who can predict, however, which antisocials will become murderously violent? Perhaps they are the ones with the most violent tendencies in childhood, repeatedly setting fires or torturing animals. Or, maybe they show, like Gacy and Ted Bundy, the most extreme deficits of conscience, leading psychologist Robert Hare and others to call them Cleckley *psychopaths*, as described in Chapter 2. To Hare, Gacy is an example of a cold-blooded, conscienceless killer who repels and fascinates us. To know Gacy is to understand both his cold and calculating rationality and his "inability to treat others as thinking, feeling human beings." Says Hare: "Such morally incomprehensible behavior, exhibited by a seemingly normal person, leaves us feeling bewildered and helpless."[11]

A late colleague, child psychiatrist Richard Jenkins, was fascinated by my study of antisocials, Gacy in particular. He told me that, in 1984, he had asked Eve Gowdey, another former colleague, to interpret Gacy's 1968 Sentence Completion Test—with Gacy's name removed, of course. The test—a list of 40 sentence fragments that the patient is asked to complete—is intended to provide clues to the patient's inner thoughts, much like the Rorschach ink blots. Gowdey's reading produced a far more chilling assessment than any found in Gacy's file. "The most striking impression," she wrote, "is the feeling this man is sorry he was caught." She went on to suspect that he was "physically and grossly aggressive to anyone he considered in his power, [and that] any change in his behavior would originate only by chance and then from something outside of himself." Finally, she stated that she would "never trust this man or expect any improvement in his behavior. I would assume [that he was] physically dangerous to anyone he thought was powerless." By then, of course, Gacy was on death row.

In some ways, Gacy's story contradicts much of what we know about the natural history of ASP. Jenkins himself theorized that one could predict outcomes of juvenile delinquency based on delinquents' socialization, that is the ability to form bonds with others. Socialized delinquents established such bonds and, in Jenkins's eyes, were less likely to continue delinquent behaviors than were their undersocialized peers. Other research indicates that children with conduct disorder who exhibit the earliest and most severe symptoms stand the greatest risk of developing adult ASP. They are also the ones most likely to perpetrate violence toward others.[12] For children and adults, psychiatric research—as well as common sense—predicts that extreme misbehavior begets further extremes, that patients who are the worst upon assessment experience the worst outcomes. Gacy, however, demonstrates that no predictive theory is flawless when confronting a disorder as complex and mysterious as ASP. Although he grew up feeling afraid and different, he was moderately well behaved and had few characteristics of delinquency, with no juvenile arrest record or early history of violence. His problems with school and petty theft deepened during his teen years but, by adulthood, Gacy was working successfully and forming relationships with those around him. In short, he seemed, for a while, at least on the surface, to have escaped the pitfalls of his early life.

PATHWAY TO MURDER

Like ASP, *serial murder* is an old phenomenon but a relatively new term, having entered the common lexicon with the reports of the rapes and murders committed by Ted Bundy in the 1970s.[13] Stories of killers like Jack the Ripper, the unknown slasher who terrorized London in the 1880s, as well as legends of vampires and werewolves—which may have originated from strings of brutal, unexplained murders— show how societies have long feared the very real monsters that lurk beyond the fringes of morality and human comprehension. In recent decades, their crimes have been classified and examined as the work of distinct criminal types, but their stories continue to take on mythic proportions, perhaps because such killers seem inhuman, oblivious to the emotions and moral reason that guide normal lives.

Michael Stone, a Columbia University psychiatrist, writes about killers in his book *The Anatomy of Evil*, and explains his system of "gradations" of evil, with serial murder at the extreme end because of its recreational nature, the associated torture, and the shear callousness of the act.[14] Carl Panzram, who admitted committing 21 murders and thousands of rapes and other crimes in the 1920s and 1930s, would certainly qualify for anchoring the extreme end of Stone's gradations. Panzram claimed to be "meanness personified" and to hate the entire human race, himself included.[15] He was an unruly child, first arrested for being drunk and disorderly at age eight, then charged with a string of robberies that sent him to a reformatory. Panzram is said to have lured a group of sailors aboard a yacht, gotten them drunk, sexually assaulted them, then killed them and dumped their bodies over the side. On a trip to Africa, he allegedly hired eight guides, whom he slaughtered and fed to crocodiles. He was finally hanged for murdering a man in prison, but denied having any remorse for his crimes.

Panzram's unrelenting viciousness, lack of conscience, perpetual status as a social outsider, and long criminal career suggest ASP. James Alan Fox and Jack Levin, criminologists at Northeastern University, who have studied serial murder, point out that most thrill-motivated serial killers—those who do not murder for jealousy, money, or revenge—meet the criteria for ASP rather than psychotic illnesses.[16] They are not legally insane and can tell the difference between right and wrong in an intellectual sense, but they lack the emotional connection to morality that keeps most people in line. Fox and Levin point out that some serial killers murder for reasons other than thrills, such as the desire to further a cause or to collect money. They also maintain that many serial killers display some level of social conformity, fit into their communities, like Gacy, or, like Jeffrey Dahmer, need to dehumanize their victims somehow before killing them.

Regardless of their differences in method, motive, or mental status, many serial killers share a history of behavior problems—some mild, others severe—that indicate possible ASP. Nearly all serial killers exhibit antisocial tendencies that may be seen, if only in retrospect, as precursors to murderous behavior. Ted Bundy was an isolated and insecure child but also a pathological liar, shoplifter, thief, and window peeper.[17] A former law student, the handsome and well spoken Bundy led a hideous secret life, mutilating his victims, having sex with their corpses, even suffocating a little girl by shoving her face in the mud. Danny Rolling, who butchered five college students in Gainesville, Florida, had a history of theft, robbery, and assault, and once attempted to kill his own father.[18] Robert Hansen began having trouble with the law during childhood and was at various times a shoplifter, robber, arsonist, and violent assailant.[19] Also an avid hunter, Hansen lost interest in conventional game and began kidnapping women, whom he would set loose and hunt down in the Alaska woods.

Some serial killers come from backgrounds of savage abuse and deprivation, perhaps born to parents who are themselves antisocial. Henry Lee Lucas was the son of an alcoholic father who lost his legs under a freight train and a mother who reportedly had sex with men while making Henry watch. She beat her son with pieces of lumber and assorted other weapons, told him he was evil and would eventually die in prison, and sent him to school dressed like a girl, his hair curled into ringlets. Lucas claimed she killed his pet mule with a shotgun, part of her ongoing effort to destroy his every source of pleasure. By his teens, Lucas had suffered serious head trauma and lost an eye that his brother accidentally punctured with a knife. He was also stealing money and food, and catching small animals that he skinned alive. He claimed to have committed his first murder at age 15, when a rape attempt went awry, and that year was sent to a reformatory for breaking and entering. His life became a series of arrests, convictions, and jail sentences, including a 40-year term for second-degree murder after he fatally stabbed his mother. He was paroled from a Michigan prison in 1970, despite warning officials that he would kill again. Over the next 13 years, he kept his word, later claiming to have committed hundreds of murders along a 500-mile stretch of interstate highway running from Texas to Florida. His alleged victims included children, women young and old, middle-aged businessmen, hitchhikers, vagrants, and even his 14-year-old common-law wife, whom he stabbed, raped, and cut into pieces. Asked why he would do such a thing to one he claimed to love, Lucas responded, "It was the only thing I could think of."[20]

Although abuse and its lifelong physical and emotional scars are often part of a killer's background, they explain neither serial murder nor ASP. Purported causes of serial murder—including abuse, brain injury, various forms of psychosis, and even ASP—do not apply to every case. Jeffrey Dahmer, the Milwaukee man who killed and dismembered 17 young men and boys, seemed to have had a relatively peaceful childhood, albeit one dominated by bizarre fantasies and obsessions.[21] Although some sketchy reports of parental abuse and neglect surfaced after his arrest for murder, they pale next to the stories of men like Henry Lucas, as does Dahmer's scant record of youthful misbehavior. He grew up a loner, indulging his hobbies of dissecting small animals that he killed or found dead by the road, but largely staying out of trouble. He later developed a chronic drinking problem while in the Army and was discharged. As a young man, he drew police attention for disorderly conduct, indecent exposure, and child sex abuse, and was nearly caught when a 14-year-old boy ran naked and bleeding from his apartment. But police who confronted Dahmer believed his claim that he and the youth were lovers and sent the boy back to his death. Only when another would-be victim escaped did authorities discover the killing chamber that Dahmer's home had become. Photos of murdered men adorned its walls, a 55-gallon drum contained a soup of acid and human remains, and severed heads were stored in the refrigerator and freezer, along with a human heart preserved for a later meal.

One challenge of studying any antisocial is the constant need to evaluate critically what he says, separating fact from fiction. Some murderers, like Lucas, admit to crimes they did not commit, whereas others, like Gacy, make a sustained effort to deny responsibility for their actions. Before being sentenced for his murder conviction, Dahmer told the court, "I ask for no consideration. I know my time in prison will be terrible. But I deserve whatever I get because of what I have done."[22] He apologized to his family, the families of his victims, and the police officers who had been fired for returning a young boy to Dahmer's deadly hands. Who can say whether Dahmer truly regretted his crimes, whether he had finally realized that what he did was terribly wrong? He had certainly proven himself an accomplished liar, able to deceive his victims and the police. Such admissions of guilt could indicate a glimmer of conscience, but they could just as likely be last-ditch efforts to beg for the court's mercy.

Dahmer's confessions and apparent need to dehumanize his victims—by attempting to turn some into zombielike sex slaves through crude "lobotomies," in which he drilled holes into their skulls—led Fox and Levin to argue that he displayed a modicum of conscience and was thus not a "true sociopath." Indeed, serial murderers may be driven by a range of mental problems, from personality disorders to genuine psychosis. Ed Gein, a Wisconsin farmer who robbed graves and eventually murdered women in order to craft for himself a suit of human skin (his story influenced films from *Psycho* to *Silence of the Lambs*), was apparently insane.[23] But killers who know right from wrong, who kill repeatedly without remorse, and whose histories are marked by other incidents of antisocial behavior raise the suspicion of ASP. Applying psychiatric diagnoses to crimes that involve incomprehensible brutality, however, is a challenge, involving not only the intricacies of diagnosis itself, but also its implications for criminal prosecution, defense, and punishment.

Another challenge to those who study serial murder is to explain why so few women are in their ranks—but, then again, we have few clues as to why ASP primarily occurs in men.[24] One of the few well-publicized cases of a woman serial murderer is that of Aileen Wuernos, portrayed by actress Charlize Theron in the highly praised film *Monster*. Executed in Florida in 2002 for the murder of seven men between 1989 and 1990, Wuernos claimed the men had raped or attempted to rape her while she worked as a prostitute. Wuernos, who grew up in a severely abusive family, began her life of crime early, offering sex in exchange for cigarettes, drugs, or food at age 11. Over the following decades, she was arrested multiple times on a range of charges, including prostitution, assault, forgery, and armed robbery, and spent considerable time incarcerated. In 1991, she was arrested in a sting operation, after her female lover got her to confess to murder during a series of monitored phone calls, in exchange for prosecutorial immunity. In the end, Wuernos received six death sentences. She petitioned the Florida Supreme Court to end all appeals that others were filing in her behalf, saying "I killed those men, robbed them cold as ice. I'd do it again, too."[25]

THE TRIAL OF GACY

Out of prison and back in Chicago, Gacy began working as a cook and making plans for a fresh start. His first wife had divorced him during his prison stay, taking with her the children and most of their joint property. In fact, all that remained for Gacy was his movie camera, projector, screen, and the pornographic films seized from their home in Waterloo. Gacy's father had died while his son was behind bars, so John moved into his mother's condo until he could persuade her to loan him money for the house at 8213 Summerdale, where they continued to live together. By this time, Gacy had left restaurant work to begin his own contracting business. He had also become reacquainted with a high school friend who had been through a divorce of her own. They dated for seven months, then married. When she and her two daughters moved into the house, there was already a body buried in the crawl space, just below the bedroom she shared with her new husband.

Less than a year after his release from prison, Gacy had been charged for assaulting a teenage boy, who reported that Gacy tried to force him to engage in sex after picking him up at the Greyhound bus station. Again, Gacy tried to blame the victim, alleging that he had thrown the boy out of his car to rebuff a sexual advance. In a tragic turn of events, the case was dismissed when the boy failed to appear in court. It was never reported to the Iowa parole board, and the next boy Gacy met at the bus station, on January 2, 1972, was not so fortunate. Years later, a coroner's report would state that this first unidentified victim died of stab wounds, which Gacy would claim resulted from either an accident or self-defense. Remarkably, Gacy escaped a number of other close brushes with the law, including an incident nine days before his wedding that brought an arrest for aggravated battery and reckless conduct involving another young man picked up on the Chicago streets. It never went to trial. Two other young men filed complaints against Gacy during his years of murder, one even pursuing his case in a civil suit alleging that Gacy had kidnapped and repeatedly raped him during a terrifying night in early 1978. But none of the allegations was taken seriously until Gacy was charged with more than 30 killings, perhaps because some of Gacy's accusers were openly gay men.

Just as he had in Waterloo, Gacy managed to keep his secret life hidden from those around him, including his wife. Again, things seemed normal on the surface as Gacy plunged into his work and gradually developed his meager contracting business into a growing enterprise. He volunteered with the Democratic Party, became its local precinct captain, and joined the Moose Lodge, where he discovered a new love. Wearing makeup and outfits of his own design, Gacy took the name Pogo and joined the lodge's Jolly Joker Clown Club, entertaining children and quelling his own demons. "Pogo was a tranquilizer," Gacy would say. "When I was Pogo, I was in another world."[26] Perhaps only professional clowns would realize a mistake Gacy made in his makeup: While most clowns paint their mouths with rounded corners so as not to frighten children, Gacy drew his with sharp points.

The semblance of normalcy began to fade as Gacy's second marriage soured. Once an engaging companion to his wife and a kind provider for her children, Gacy stepped up his drinking and began popping pills to help him sleep or to boost him through long days. His behavior became erratic, punctuated by fits of temper that his wife came to fear. Their sexual life dwindled until Gacy declared it over. Although he had told her that he was bisexual before they married, she had never regarded his sexuality as a threat until she found a cache of homosexual pornography and evidence of his masturbation. She began to suspect that he found sexual outlets in the young men with whom he spent so much time, some of them employees, others strangers. They divorced, and Gacy was left alone in the house.

Only months before his final arrest, Gacy passed a security clearance that permitted him to meet the First Lady after a parade he had organized. He hosted his annual yard party, cooking for wealthy clients and politicians who had no way of knowing about the body concealed under the backyard barbecue pit. But after his final victim disappeared, the boy's parents urged the police to pursue Gacy, who they knew was the last person to see him. The police uncovered Gacy's record of previous offenses involving young men. Under interrogation, Gacy realized he was caught, but his demeanor never changed. As one investigator described it:

> It finally dawned on him that it was over. The game he was playing, this dual life he was leading, was finally exposed. But he still thought he would call the shots. He was like "O.K., we are going to clear up thirty-some murders." He was smoking cigars and he was the center of attention with six or seven people interviewing him. In his mind that made him a big deal. Mr. Big-Shot. He never showed any emotion. I cannot emphasize this enough. He has never in my dealings with him showed one ounce of remorse or sorrow or sympathy.[27]

Although he talked, Gacy frustrated police investigators and his own attorneys by claiming to remember only a few of the murders. His details were ambiguous, including theories about how various victims might have upset him or otherwise precipitated their own deaths. He also suggested that a brutish alter ego might have been responsible for the killings. During the six-week trial, Gacy's attorneys argued that he was not guilty by reason of insanity and should be institutionalized rather than imprisoned or executed.[28] The prosecution, on the other hand, presented evidence that the killings were premeditated and that Gacy was a sadistic, cold-blooded murderer fully aware of what he was doing. After all, he had instructed his employees to excavate trenches in the crawl space, giving careful instructions about where to dig and which areas to avoid. The defense called a series of psychiatric experts to testify that Gacy suffered from a mental illness that caused him to swing from periods of normalcy to intense psychosis. One called Gacy a "pseudo-neurotic paranoid schizophrenic" whose mental illness stemmed from childhood abuse by his father. Another testified that he had "borderline personality organization with a subtype of antisocial or psychopathic personality manifested by episodes of an underlying condition of paranoid schizophrenia." Additional testimony depicted Gacy as paranoid, obsessive, narcissistic, "polymorphously perverse," and fearful of his sexuality. Despite their differences, the defense experts all agreed that Gacy's was a complex case and that his murderous acts were the product of a deep-seated and uncontrollable condition that met the legal conditions for insanity.[29]

The prosecution conducted a skeptical cross-examination and rebutted with its own string of psychiatric experts. The first was Leonard Heston, the psychiatrist who had evaluated Gacy at the University of Iowa in 1968. He told the court that Gacy had been diagnosed with ASP after his sodomy charge and was thus considered sane at the time. Although he agreed with a defense witness's observation that Gacy displayed antisocial traits, he condemned much of the preceding testimony as "six or eight terms that are all thrown in a pudding." He added that subjects with personality disorders do not display the psychosis that Gacy's defense team aimed to prove. A second expert agreed that Gacy had a "psychopathic or antisocial personality with sexual deviation" and said he saw no evidence that Gacy had ever lost the capacity to understand that his conduct was wrong. He was not psychotic. Instead, he continued, Gacy was deliberately evasive, misleading, and intent on rationalizing his actions—all hallmarks of ASP.

The third prosecution expert directly stated that he thought Gacy was lying during his examination and that Gacy was driven by a personality disorder, either narcissistic or antisocial. He did not believe Gacy had suffered 33 separate instances of temporary insanity, and he thought Gacy's methods—the calculating steps he took to lure young men home with him, sometimes tricking them into putting on handcuffs—showed he was never out of touch with reality while committing his crimes. Gacy's effort to attribute the murders to an alternate personality was simply part of a transparent plot to fake insanity. The final expert for the state weighed in with a diagnosis of "mixed personality disorder" that combined narcissistic and antisocial elements. In the most damning statement yet, he argued that Gacy's condition would probably not meet the state's involuntary commitment statute, and that Gacy would eventually have to be released from a psychiatric hospital if sent there rather than to prison.

At this point, Gacy protested to the judge that he had opposed the insanity defense adopted by his lawyers, but the trial continued with more experts, this time testifying for the defense and the notion that Gacy was psychotic. The prosecution continued to attack their assessments during cross-examination and brought in yet another expert to disagree with the defense's theory of insanity. Prosecutors closed by stating that Gacy was evil. His defense team argued that "he was eaten up by his raging illness." After less than two hours of deliberation, the jury sided with the prosecution, finding John Wayne Gacy guilty of murder. The next day, they sentenced him to death. Only after 14 years and several failed appeals was Gacy finally executed, on May 10, 1994, the 26th anniversary of his first arrest in Iowa.

The Gacy story doesn't end there. His artwork—usually paintings of clowns—occasionally shows up for sale on eBay, and the process of identifying his victims continues. As recently as November 2011, another victim, who had remained nameless for more than three decades, was identified through the science of DNA testing, to the great relief of his family members.[30]

CONFRONTING THE KILLERS

About half of the psychiatrists and psychologists who took the stand during Gacy's trial declared that his disorder was one of personality or character rather than true insanity. Based on what I have learned about the case, I fully agree. Gacy had shown an antisocial streak since childhood, although his early behavior problems were relatively minor—truancy, poor school performance, and occasional shoplifting. As an adult, Gacy showed signs of ASP in his elaborate con jobs, blatant lying, physical assaults and, ultimately, murders. Nevertheless, he continued to work successfully and remain active in community life. Gacy was indeed a complex personality, and it is possible that therapy might have helped him overcome his troublesome childhood memories and sexual distress. But in all his dealings with mental health professionals, Gacy displayed an attitude of superiority and indifference to his problems. He seemed to think himself smarter than his doctors, able to lie his way through their tests and manipulate their diagnoses.

John Douglas, a former FBI agent and an expert on serial killers, warns that mental health professionals must be wary when evaluating serial murderers: "Often, [professionals] don't understand that in trying to assess these convicts, they're actually assessing individuals who are themselves expert in assessing people!"[31] Psychiatrists and psychologists are trained to suspect when a patient is lying or trying to simulate serious mental illness, but they sometimes make mistakes. They may also be driven by idealistic notions of treatment to overlook the reality of ASP and to see improvement where none has occurred.

Virtually all psychiatrists agree that antisocials must be considered accountable for their actions, but lawyers may see ASP and other personality disorders as a potential defense for their clients.[32] In truth, antisocials fail the legal tests designed to pardon defendants who are truly psychotic. The basis for the legal notion of insanity in many states is the so-called *M'Naghten* rule—named for the man who, in 1843, shot and killed the British prime minister's personal secretary after experiencing delusions for several years. It holds that persons seeking the insanity defense must show that their mental illness was so extreme they were unable to know the nature and quality of the act, or were unable to know it was wrong. Because antisocials know the difference between right and wrong, ASP alone is simply not a sufficient basis for supporting an insanity defense. Those with ASP realize their behavior runs contrary to the law, but they just don't seem to care.

Successful insanity defenses are rare, usually succeeding only in cases where defendants are clearly out of touch with reality—like serial killer Ed Gein, who spent 27 years in a hospital for the criminally insane. Gacy's trial demonstrates that expert witnesses called to testify may offer a variety of psychiatric rationales for a defendant's behavior—some based on legitimate professional differences, others on unscrupulous money-grubbing. Witnesses, attorneys, judges, and the men and women who make up juries must realize that excusing antisocials on false grounds can have disastrous effects. If released from custody, they stand a strong chance of committing further crimes. If confined to hospitals, they strain the mental health care system, often cause trouble, and are unlikely to improve. Although antisocials scoff at standards of all kinds, they clearly have the intellectual capacity to make moral judgments but simply lack the emotional will to do so. They must therefore be held responsible for their actions, as the threat of punishment sometimes becomes a deterrent that replaces their absent moral sense. The desire to evade responsibility is a facet of ASP itself, and excusing antisocials for their misbehavior simply promotes their disorder.

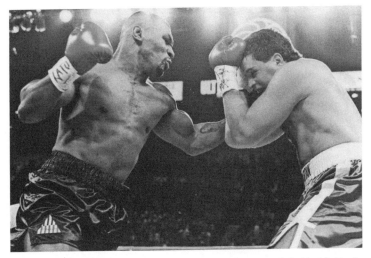

Boxing champion Mike Tyson's (on left) antisocial behavior has provided tabloid fodder for nearly three decades (Getty Images).

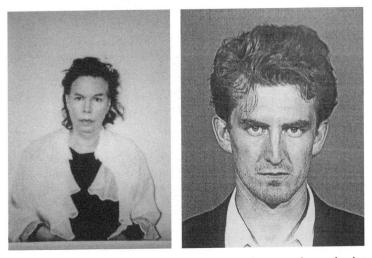

Sante and Kenneth Kimes were notorious for their mother/son criminal escapades that included murder (Getty Images).

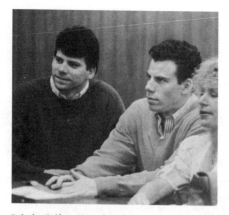

Lyle (on left) and Eric (right) Menendez admitted to killing their parents but blamed it on years of physical and sexual abuse (Getty Images).

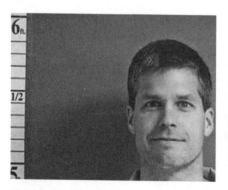

Alex Kelly's wealthy family was unable to keep him out of prison (Getty Images).

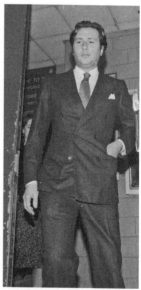

The handsome Raffaelo Follieri was known as the "Vati-con" for his claim of being close to the Pope (Getty Images).

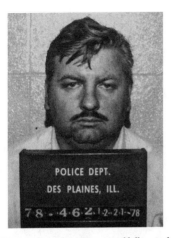

John Wayne Gacy, one of America's most notorious serial killers, is shown here in a mug shot, though he often appears in photos as his alter ego, Pogo the Clown (Getty Images).

John Gacy NO0921
Lock Box 711
Menard, Illinois 62259
May 28th, 1989

Sorry to disappoint you, and I don't know where you got the information. I have enclosed a copy of the typical route of a capital case on Appeal. The news media just likes to see my name in print, or they are hard up for news. In any case my appeal just finished step number four, so you can read on from there.

Regarding any interviews, those request go through my attorney or agent in New York, the fee is $500.00 a minute for the first hour which has to be paid in advance for the first hour, and the money goes to charity. It is the same kind of fees doctors are paid for being professional witnesses, and just as unreliable as to what will be said, according to whos side they are on.

Have a nice day.

Best regards,

J W GACY

John Wayne Gacy

cc/ file People up to no good.

This was Gacy's letter to us declining study participation in our follow-up study of antisocial men (Collection of Donald W. Black).

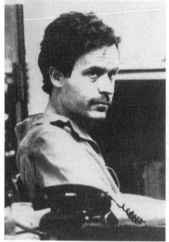

Former law student Ted Bundy represented himself in court in a Florida murder case in 1978 (Getty Images).

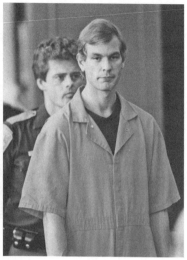

Jeffrey Dahmer is known for having cannibalized many of his victims (Getty Images).

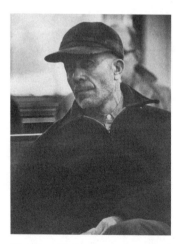

Ed Gein robbed graves and murdered women, but was probably insane (Getty Images).

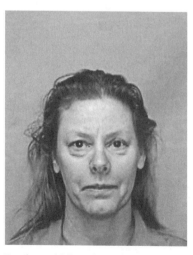

Female serial killer Aileen Wuernos was portrayed in the blockbuster movie *Monster* (Getty Images).

Chapter 10

Antisocial Personality Disorder and Families

Finding Ways to Cope

THE PROBLEM HAS A NAME

Antisocial personality disorder (ASP) is not a sudden development, not a quiet condition that ticks away beneath the surface of normal life before one day exploding. Rather, it is a looming presence that seldom escapes notice by those nearby. Every antisocial leaves a trail of disruption, deceit, and even violence that begins early in life, and every antisocial family comes to recognize the symptoms of ASP, even if they fail to see them as part of a long-term pattern. For many, learning that the problem has a name brings new hope for change.

But discovery is only the beginning. Whether or not the antisocial seeks professional help, his family members must respond to the disorder, a process that sometimes comes down to a clear but difficult decision—to leave an antisocial relative or to stay and learn to cope. Antisocials cannot be forced to change. The drive to get better and to find a new way of relating to the world must come from within, although family members can exert a valuable influence and provide much-needed support. Even as an antisocial considers his tumultuous history of behavior and assesses his desire for change, family members must take a long, hard look at themselves and their relationships with him. What they find may cause surprise or dismay and may lead to understanding, strength, or the desire to escape.

Many of the case studies in this book include brief accounts of family members caught in the web of ASP. Jim (from Chapter 5), the man who attacked Cathy when she tried to interview him, had been married to a woman who stuck by him as he descended into alcoholism. She told his doctors that she remembered his good side and how her support had enabled him to go to college, marry, and leave his bad times behind. When the problems returned and their relationship soured, she remained steadfast in her resolve to see him through. Although she could not imagine leaving him, she later sought a divorce when staying became too difficult. Edward's parents

(Chapter 3) likewise clung to hope in the face of constant disappointment. Whenever their son disappeared or got into trouble with the law, they would welcome him back with encouragement and the irresistible magnet of money. Their efforts to buy his way out of trouble and into a respectable life failed, and Ed's brother remembered their mistakes in his hard-nosed refusal to help. He loved his brother but had seen how Ed manipulated and took advantage of his parents, giving nothing in return.

Family responses to an ASP diagnosis vary greatly, from relief to anger. Those who have tried to help a relative overcome years of bad decisions and frustrating behavior may feel intense guilt when they learn how they might have enabled him to continue on his course. Even then, they may find it difficult to stop covering his tracks. Others deny the problem altogether, sometimes focusing on specific symptoms of the disorder or arguing that it will pass on its own. For some family members, it is easier to attribute bad behavior to alcoholism or a spell of unemployment than to a serious personality disorder. Richard's wife (Chapter 8), for example, insisted there was nothing wrong with her husband aside from his immaturity—even though he had just been hospitalized after drinking a bottle of rubbing alcohol. Still others may see the diagnosis as a license to leave the relationship, the end of a disturbing chapter in their lives that can finally be explained. The fact that many antisocials have other family members with the disorder or tend to marry spouses with antisocial traits can produce fear, denial, or the desire for escape. "If he is antisocial," family members may wonder, "what does that make me?"

The general lack of knowledge about ASP and the perplexing nature of personality disorders in general make an ASP diagnosis uncharted territory for most family members forced to confront the disorder. They most likely have not heard of it, or they may wrongly think it has something to do with disliking social situations. The psychiatric literature can be as disturbing as it is informative—that is, assuming family members are willing to wade through pages of jargon and scientific analysis. Words like *sociopath* and *psychopath* carry frightening connotations, which is one reason I prefer the term *antisocial*. Any major psychiatric diagnosis should come from a mental health professional who can clearly and simply explain how the disorder is identified, what it means, and what to expect. Information is essential if family members are to confront the disorder and become partners in therapy, especially when the outlook is grim.

ADVICE FOR FAMILIES

As Cleckley put it more than 70 years ago in *The Mask of Sanity*, "If a proper general understanding could be reached that psychopaths have a serious psychiatric abnormality and are not likely under prevailing conditions to become better, and if this fact could be disseminated, their families might be able to reconcile themselves better to a major problem and seek more realistic ways of dealing with it."[1] My hope in this book is to offer some of that understanding, especially for people who live with ASP every day, either in themselves or in someone they love. Toward that end, my advice to families of antisocials has six basic elements:

Accept the diagnosis. Family members must come to grips with the disorder and acknowledge that ASP exists, even when the antisocial does not. They must realize the disorder will not go away and, even with a concerted effort, improvement may take years fraught with the constant threat of relapse. Some antisocials will insist that mental health professionals keep the diagnosis a secret under the guise of confidentiality. A good psychiatrist or psychologist will respond by emphasizing that family members have an essential role in treatment. Once they know, family members should learn all they can about the disorder, preferably firsthand from a professional. They can also read about ASP, although relatively few books are available for lay or even professional audiences (some are recommended at the end of this book). As they learn about the nature of ASP, many will find that pieces of the puzzle suddenly fall into place and that their experiences with this difficult disorder are not unique, which can be reassuring.

Urge treatment. Although the antisocial patient must develop insight and get serious about therapy on his own, having close relatives behind him makes it all the more likely that he will pursue treatment and then stay the course. Family members use different strategies to encourage the process, usually before they realize that the problem is ASP. Many focus on a single issue—alcoholism, uncontrolled anger, depression, or relationship problems—that is easier for the "patient" to recognize. This problem becomes the chief complaint when an antisocial is assessed by a mental health professional, and it is the stepping stone to an ASP diagnosis. Wives sometimes resort to the threat of divorce if their spouses do not seek help. Although they can be effective, threats are a risky gambit that should not be undertaken without careful thought, as they may backfire or even provoke violence. When an antisocial sees a threat not followed through, he gains confidence and another tool for manipulation. Conversely, laying down a firm bottom line may be the final jab that brings an antisocial to recognize his problems. An antisocial man who hears his wife say "See a doctor or I'm leaving" and knows she means it might finally get the message.

Be firm with children. Taking a stand against antisocial behavior can be hard for parents, no matter what age their children are. The impulse to protect one's offspring at any cost makes some parents, even those of adult antisocials, incapable of being firm in the face of their children's misbehavior. Parents of teenagers and young children with severe behavior problems—the type that may develop into adult ASP—face especially difficult challenges since their children cannot be cut off financially or kicked out of the house as a last resort. Nevertheless, a "tough love" stance may be most effective. Antisocials and children with conduct disorder must learn that they are responsible for their own behavior and accept the consequences of their actions. They must see that their days of manipulating parents and family members are over and that they have to make an effort to change. Studies have shown that special training for parents may be the best weapon for fighting conduct disorder in young children.[2] By learning the appropriate parenting skills they need to stop misbehavior before it escalates into violence, parents may help reduce their children's risk of ASP later in life. Parents of older children can learn similar coping skills from therapists but above all should realize their essential role in advocating right behavior and standing up to wrong.

Protect yourself from abuse. When abuse enters a relationship, the best response is to get out fast. Antisocials have a dangerous proclivity for verbal, physical, or sexual mistreatment, taking out their frustrations on spouses, partners, children, or parents. No one deserves abuse, but some victims feel they have asked for it or that things might get better with time. That said, once abusive behavior starts, it tends not to stop, often growing worse instead. Victims of abuse should protect themselves by leaving the household or cutting off contact with the batterer, seeking protection in the home of a relative or friend or at a domestic violence shelter. Many communities have such shelters, particularly for battered women. Victims may fear revenge or other potential consequences, but leaving the abusive situation is often better than trying to survive in a relationship built on fear and violence.

Consider your motives. An ASP diagnosis forces family members to think about their relationship with the antisocial and to assess their own choices. When abuse is a factor, it is essential that victims who remain in the relationship consider why they are willing to stay. Although it may be obvious to others that the relationship is destructive, some victims—most of them women—choose to suffer through it for reasons they do not understand. Some have come to believe the insults hurled at them or to feel they deserve punishment. Others are unaware that they are being abused, especially by a manipulative and controlling antisocial partner. They may think abuse is a natural part of a relationship, especially if they come from families in which violence or verbal assaults were common. With the encouragement of a therapist, victims of abuse can come to understand their choices and learn to be more confident and assertive. Support groups for battered spouses or family members of alcoholics (Al-Anon is one well-known organization) can be extremely helpful, introducing a person to others who have lived with antisocial behavior. Family members of antisocials—especially those who have experienced abuse—should seek out these groups and the help they offer.

Recognize that it's not your fault. Those close to an antisocial must understand that they did not cause his problems. They should resist blaming themselves, which can be extremely hard to do. Parents especially may find themselves unable to stop second-guessing their decisions and searching for something they may have done wrong. (The exception, of course, is the abusive parent who may well have contributed to the child's antisocial behavior.) Although relatives and friends of an antisocial need to think about how their behavior might influence him, they also should realize that his disorder is deeply rooted and beyond their control. Likewise, they should not hold themselves responsible if treatment fails.

THE THREAT OF DOMESTIC VIOLENCE

The threat of domestic violence remains all too common. Antisocials are at particularly high risk for committing violent acts directed at their partners or children.[3] Many antisocials become abusive at some point in their relationships—whether hurling insults, restricting their partners' freedom, striking out with fists, or even raping their partners. No amount of media coverage and public discussion will eliminate what remains largely a private nightmare, and every victim of abuse must decide when to call on others for help. Fortunately, more resources exist for abuse victims than ever before, and law enforcement agencies are increasingly prepared to treat domestic violence like the crime it is.

Women are the most frequent victims of domestic violence and men the most common perpetrators, although the roles are occasionally reversed (domestic violence occurs in gay and lesbian relationships, as well). The goal of domestic violence is control, usually through escalating stages of abusive behavior that begin with intimidation. An abusive man may attempt to isolate his female partner from her friends and family, control how she spends her time, or force unwanted sexual relations. He may try emotional blackmail, perhaps threatening to kidnap or hurt the woman's children. Finally, he may threaten to do her physical harm or even to kill her. Isolated incidents of physical violence may become a steady trickle that builds over years if the relationship continues.

Some victims of domestic violence remain in dysfunctional relationships even as violence becomes more common. In *Shot in the Heart*, Mikal Gilmore reflects on why his mother, Bessie, stayed with his abusive, antisocial father:

> My mother's failure to leave my father was not a unique thing. People stay in bad relationships all the time—women stay with men who hurt them emotionally and physically and men stay with women who berate them or shut them out. Sometimes you stay because you love the person, and you can't imagine life without looking at that lover's face. Maybe you hope things will improve. Maybe the love blinds you—maybe you don't know you're being abused. [When asked why she put up with the

beatings,] especially the ones that left her face knotted with ugly black lumps and bruises, "Hell," she said, "I asked for all that...I deserved it." It's as simple as that.[4]

Abused partners stay for many reasons, some understood only by themselves. They may be unable to conceive any alternatives or may have strong feelings for the abusive partner, despite the violence. They may see no financial alternative. Some stay out of concern for their children, but they, too, are usually better off outside the abusive home, especially when they are potential victims. Some victims are further troubled by health problems, mental illness, or addictions that bind them to the batterer.

Patterns of abuse are shaped by the dynamics of each relationship, and sometimes both partners contribute to the cycle, especially when both tend toward antisocial behavior or have trouble with intimacy. He assaults, and she responds by provoking his anger or jealousy. He assaults again, and the two become locked in a dance of destruction that slowly escalates as the relationship becomes increasingly unstable. More commonly, the abused partner does not provoke mistreatment but simply does little to stop it. When the batterer suspects that she is turning for help outside the home, he may commit a flurry of assaults in a last-ditch effort to keep control. He will refuse counseling, insisting she is at fault and criticizing her for bringing outsiders into their relationship. Protecting oneself and finding help is the best response to an abusive situation.

Taking a strong stand and ending the relationship is the best way to leave abuse behind, but it takes enormous courage. The abused partner must break any lingering ties to the batterer while fighting the fear that he may seek revenge, driven by raw anger and the sense that he has been abandoned. Although leaving is the best escape, the decision to do so will sometimes place the victim in greater danger and therefore requires careful thought. Factors like money, housing, and the safety of children must enter the equation. Legal options must be considered. When an abused partner decides she has had enough, her plan should be worked out in advance: a change of clothes hidden in the car, an extra set of car keys made, a place to stay arranged, and access to a phone. Simple details like the batterer's car blocking the driveway can destroy an otherwise sound plan. When there is immediate cause for concern, or if the abuser learns of the plan, the fleeing victim may want to call the police.

The law can offer assistance, often in the form of restraining (or protective) orders that require the abuser to keep his distance. These orders generally require some proof of assault involving physical violence, threat with a dangerous weapon, or threat of immediate harm. Protective orders are sometimes called *no-contact* orders. When they come during a divorce, paternity case, or custody proceedings, they are known as *restraining orders* or *injunctions*. Each has its own rules, but all aim to prevent violence. When an abuser violates the rules, perhaps showing up at a victim's residence or threatening and harassing her, the police can be called to arrest him. A 1994 federal law also makes batterers who violate no-contact orders subject to losing their firearms.[5] When children are involved, judges may award temporary custody to abused partners, sometimes determining visitation, support arrangements, and use of the family home. This is a prelude to divorce when the couple is married, but many abused partners return to the relationship and ask that the orders be rescinded.

Abused partners who remain on their own must learn how to protect themselves with help from the law and local resources. Protective orders and threats of jail keep some men away, but others—including many antisocials—see legal documents as meaningless scraps of paper that do nothing more than document the batterer's loss and, in his eyes, the invasion of authority into his private affairs. Court orders do not guarantee safety, but they are an improvement over old laws that required a victim to experience more serious assault before filing a complaint. Attorneys can help obtain protective orders, but abused partners can usually get them without hiring a lawyer. Procedures vary from state to state, but the first step typically involves filing a petition for an order with the clerk of court's office in a county where either the victim or the abuser lives. The abused partner must describe her relationship with the batterer and generally is required to pay a small filing fee that may be waived if money is tight. A judge reviews the petition and decides whether to grant temporary orders, which may not go into effect until the local sheriff notifies the abuser. A copy of the order goes to area law enforcement officers, and a hearing is scheduled for both sides to present their cases. If the batterer does not show up, the abused partner may get a permanent order by default. Cases are sometimes settled out of court if lawyers represent both sides.

In most states, domestic battery is a crime, and physical injuries are generally not necessary to file charges. Police are often required to take the abuser into custody when they receive a report of domestic violence, and they may also help the victim find a safe place to stay. For the antisocial batterer, criminal prosecution may demonstrate that abuse will not be tolerated and that his partner is serious about ending the violence. But it may also signify an intrusion that leaves the batterer deeply resentful of both his partner and the police. Convicted abusers are typically jailed or fined and, in many states, ordered to attend a batterers' program that aims to change attitudes and behavior. Needless to say, antisocials may be the most difficult batterers to educate since many have grown up in abusive households and do not care what anyone else has to say about their actions.

In *The Batterer: A Psychological Profile*, psychologist Donald Button describes follow-up studies of treated and untreated abusers, showing that violence is clearly reduced by treatment.[6] He acknowledges that treatment has little impact on some men and can actually intensify an abusive man's anger while exposing him to new ways of intimidating or physically battering his partners. However, although one-size-fits-all programs to combat abuse do not replace treatment for ASP, they remain important in the absence of any viable alternatives.

Help is available for victims of abuse, who may turn first to clergy, a therapist, a psychologist, or a psychiatrist. These professionals can offer supportive counseling, help an abused partner think about her options, and direct her to local resources. Many states have domestic abuse programs and telephone hotlines, and victims should learn what they can about area service organizations and law enforcement agencies. It is a good idea to keep phone numbers for hotlines, police, and local domestic abuse organizations in a safe place so that they are available in case of an emergency. Mental health organizations also offer assistance, and many communities have support groups and shelters specifically for victims of domestic violence.

Several national information and referral centers handle domestic violence calls from male and female victims, as well as from their abusers: the National Domestic Violence Hotline (800-799-SAFE), the Domestic Violence Hotline (800-621-HOPE), the National Center for Victims of Crime (800-FYI-CALL), the National Coalition Against Domestic Violence (303-839-1852), and the National Organization for Victims Assistance (800-879-6682). These organizations can help put victims in touch with local resources and provide relief from the torment of abuse.

OTHER CHALLENGES FOR FAMILIES

Abusive antisocials may lash out at anyone in the family, including siblings, parents, and children, and all have recourse to local law enforcement and social service organizations. Many states have passed strict laws dealing with the abuse of children and elderly dependents, who are among the most vulnerable victims. Children may be removed from the home when there is evidence of violence, however slight, although some do fall through the cracks and suffer years of physical and emotional harm. The impact of ASP on children is one of the most destructive legacies of the disorder. Countless studies have shown that the various symptoms of ASP—battery, alcoholism, poverty brought on by joblessness and irresponsibility—can echo through generations, as can the entire spectrum of symptoms that make up the disorder itself. Although hereditary factors may place children of antisocials at greater risk for ASP, environmental influences likely steer its development while placing children in serious danger as they grow up. Spouses, partners, and other relatives should consider these threats to children when pondering what to do in the wake of an ASP diagnosis.

Economic hardship often accompanies ASP, as many antisocials refuse to work, repeatedly lose jobs, or end up in prison. Men like Ernie, profiled in Chapter 2, let their spouses and children search for an income while they laze around the house or at a neighborhood bar. Alcoholism, drug addiction, compulsive gambling, and irresponsible spending can be a tremendous drain on family resources. Many community mental health organizations provide services on a sliding fee scale for low-income clients, but treatment for ASP is long, difficult, and sometimes expensive. Families of antisocials may find themselves drawing on a wide range of public resources, from Food Stamps and rental assistance to free legal aid and community child care. Financial demands alone are sometimes an incentive for family members of antisocials to strike out on their own, leaving behind the father, son, or spouse who is unable or unwilling to grapple with his disorder. Help is available, and a good therapist can advise families on where to turn for a variety of services.

Confronting ASP is more painful and difficult for family members than for antisocials themselves, as people with the disorder generally resist the notion that anything is wrong with them. The choices that families make after diagnosis depend on many things besides safety and money. Learning that a loved one has ASP can test an entire family's psychological, spiritual, and emotional strength. I wish I could say that most families come out of the experience with tighter bonds and firmer resolve to see life's challenges through but, unfortunately, this disorder brings few happy endings. It is hard but not impossible to deal with ASP, and doing so is a long-term proposition. Although mental health professionals and others can become guides, the rocky terrain of ASP is one that families must ultimately chart for themselves.

TO THE ANTISOCIAL

In the end, what happens after an ASP diagnosis is up to the antisocial himself. (The advice applies equally to women antisocials.) He can make the decision to pursue therapy or to continue his haphazard course through life, possibly losing everything in the process. For the defiant and self-absorbed antisocial, every step toward change is important, especially the initial realization that he needs help. The advice given here can make a difference, but only if the antisocial can look past his natural resistance to introspection and self-criticism—something that many refuse to do. To the antisocial serious about change, I recommend the following:

Accept that you have ASP. Coming to grips with the fact that you have the disorder is essential. After years of denying your problems and blaming others, taking a hard look at your own attitudes and behavior is not easy. But you must do it if you want to change. Realizing that you have a serious personality disorder may explain why you have made some of the choices you have, and will put you in a better position to deal with your past and your future.

Do not use ASP as an excuse to get into more trouble. Having ASP does not excuse bad behavior, nor does it stop you from making the right decisions. You are responsible for your own actions, and making up excuses for bad behavior will only hurt you. You can choose to follow the rules that everyone else follows. No one is going to let you off the hook because you have ASP, especially not the police or the courts. Antisocial personality disorder can be controlled if you are willing to do the work. If you choose not to, only you are to blame.

Use ASP as a reason to seek help. Face it—ASP makes your life harder. Knowing you have the disorder gives you a chance to make changes that can improve the rest of your life. It is very difficult to overcome ASP alone, and finding people who can help you change may have a lasting impact.

Educate yourself. Learn how ASP has affected your life, being as honest as you can about what you have done and the troubles you have encountered. Resist the urge to explain away your problems, instead recognizing them as symptoms of a disorder you can control. Talk to your doctors and counselors about ASP, and read as much as you can about it. The information is sometimes confusing or unsettling, but it can shed valuable light on your problems and help you make better decisions.

Accept that ASP is a lifelong disorder. Although ASP has been with you a long time, it is not impossible to break the hold it has over you. You didn't bring it on yourself, but you have sole responsibility for it now that it is part of your life. Don't try to blame your parents or anyone else for your ASP. The important thing is not where it comes from, but rather how you choose to deal with it.

Acknowledge how ASP has affected your family. Even though you may not have realized the severity of your behavior problems, your family no doubt has. Many people with ASP have had unhappy childhoods, have hurt their partners and children, and have broken family ties over the years. By destroying these relationships, you set yourself up for future misery. Life can be very lonely without the support of one's family, and you need family members to help you deal with ASP. Try to see things from their perspective and mend whatever relationships you can before it is too late.

A good lawyer may do you more harm than good. If you're in legal trouble, you may need an attorney, but realize that anyone who helps you escape responsibility for your actions is hurting you in the long run. No one wants to pay fines, go to jail, or be punished, but your problems come from the fact that you refuse to accept blame for what you do. When your lawyer helps you get out of trouble that you caused, understand that this does not mean that you were right to deny responsibility or to blame someone else. It may only mean that you have a good lawyer.

Try to control your temper. Getting angry brings you nothing but trouble, whether it causes a barroom brawl or a fight with your spouse. Think about how many of your problems started when you lost your temper, and how things might have been different if you had controlled your anger rather than letting it control you. Overcoming anger is one of the best things you can do to take charge of your life. A good counselor can suggest ways to defuse anger—for example, distracting yourself with an activity like exercise or taking a walk. Putting time and distance between yourself and the source of your anger can lessen the tension, but you're responsible for listening to these suggestions and making them work.

Learn to feel guilt and shame. The most important thing for you to learn is how to feel responsibility and the emotions that come with it. Most people feel bad when they do something wrong, but not you. By blaming others and creating excuses for your misbehavior, you rob yourself of the chance to learn from mistakes and to understand others. Start by accepting responsibility for your actions and realizing the impact they have on those around you. You cannot force emotions, but you can change your way of thinking so that you begin to feel them.

Learn to trust. Many people with ASP are suspicious of others' motives, making it hard for them to form and maintain strong relationships. Trust bonds people together; without it, you will continue to have trouble finding real intimacy. Learn to take words and actions at their face value, rather than searching for underlying motives, and remember that trust works both ways. As you learn to believe and accept others, you must give them reason to trust you in return.

Resist dwelling on the past. You may have been abused as a child, grown up in poverty, or seen your parents fight constantly. You may think you've had more than your share of hard times. You may even think that what you've been through justifies some of your actions or caused you to turn out the way you did. Focusing on the past makes it harder to see a future, especially when you use the past as an excuse for the present. Past events cannot be changed, but the future is in your hands.

Seek help for other problems as well. Every person with ASP brings his own set of troubles to therapy, some treatable, others not. Getting help for your ASP gives you a chance to put everything else on the table, mending relationships, overcoming addictions, and working through unresolved conflicts. Marital and family counseling, along with individual therapy, can help you attain valuable support from those closest to you. It may show you how your behavior has affected others and help family members understand you better.

If you're alcoholic or addicted to drugs, your ASP won't improve until you get these problems under control. Addiction robs you of the focus you need to fight ASP. Getting drunk or high makes it harder to judge right from wrong, to act responsibly, and to control your behavior. Complete abstinence should be your goal, and treatment should precede or coincide with therapy for ASP—either in a formal program at a hospital or clinic, or through groups like Alcoholics Anonymous.

If your doctor prescribes medication for depression, bipolar (manic-depressive) disorder, attention-deficit/hyperactivity disorder (ADHD), or some other condition, take it as directed. These disorders often complicate ASP, making it harder to control your anger, for example, or more difficult to believe you can change. There is no drug for ASP, but treating coexisting conditions with medication can help.

If you are abusing your wife, girlfriend, partner, child, parent, or anyone else, stop immediately. No one deserves your abuse, no matter what you think they may have done. It can land you in jail and destroy the relationships you need if you want to deal with ASP. With help from individual or group therapy, you can learn to overcome your anger and your need to control others. In the meantime, don't overreact if those you abuse leave or contact the police. They only want to break the cycle of battery and protect themselves. Look at their leaving as motivation to take control of your behavior.

Join support groups. Groups for antisocials do not exist, but support groups for specific symptoms—like alcoholism or domestic violence—can help you confront these particular problems. When you join a group, remember why you went and focus on listening to others. Don't become the center of attention by attacking the group's purpose or trying to justify your mistakes.

Be patient with therapy. There is no magic cure for ASP, and therapy is a learning process that takes time. Antisocials grow up without having learned some basic life skills, and it takes substantial time, effort, and concentration to make up for these losses. It's not easy, but the right therapist can help. The first therapist you see may not be the one best equipped to help you, so if your first attempt at therapy fails, try again. If you find yourself going back to old behavior patterns, don't consider the fight lost. Pick yourself up and get back on the wagon. Remember that you need to take control and that ultimately it is up to you to do so.

Antisocials may scoff at these challenges, arguing that they have complete control over their lives and don't need the help of doctors or therapists. In denying their problems, an antisocial may continue to ignore how his drinking or drug use alienates him from others, how his chronic unemployment keeps him trapped in poverty, how his lack of conscience permits him to do things others would never dream of, how his disdain for laws keeps the police on his tail. The antisocial may be completely unable to imagine a nine-to-five routine, a day without a drink, or the comfort of a meaningful relationship. Last, he may be unable to conceive that an underlying psychiatric disorder unites all his worst tendencies and that treatment can help him get better.

Men like Russ (in Chapter 7) and, to a lesser extent, Doug (in Chapter 5) improved with time, still bearing the scars of their disorder but at least able to get along in the world and to lead relatively happy lives. The bad boy who grew up to become an even worse man must find a new way of looking at the world around him and of understanding his place in society. He must accept that the rules apply to him and that he is responsible for his own behavior. He must learn to feel the emotions that most of us take for granted and to recognize those emotions in others. For many antisocials, change can happen, even if gradually, over the course of years. For them, each new gain is a milestone.

Epilogue

Dispelling the Myths

REVEALING THE MYSTERY

The antisocial's ignorance of his disorder reflects a larger misunderstanding of antisocial personality disorder (ASP) and its impact on individuals, families, and society. We are quick to attribute bad behavior to shifting social mores, poor parenting, broken families, violent video games, or countless other factors, many of which probably do influence acts and attitudes. But a look at some of the worst characters a society has to offer—career criminals, hard-core addicts, deadbeat fathers and husbands, and habitual batterers, to name a few—reveals symptoms of a psychiatric condition that has attracted notice ever since medicine began probing the mysteries of brain and mind. Blaming antisocial behavior on cultural influences and looking at isolated acts rather than patterns of behavior diverts attention from the reality of ASP. Many of the crimes and other social problems that shock and concern us can be traced in large part to a distinct group of individuals, most of them men, who act out in every conceivable way over lives filled with resentment, anger, dishonesty, violence, and moral poverty.

Examine almost any family and one will be found—the black sheep cousin, hard-drinking uncle, or con man brother. Read any newspaper, and the effects of the disorder surface—abandoned children, swindled widows, bloody assaults, even serial murder. Visit any country, society, or ethnic group, no matter how remote, and ASP becomes evident in those individuals who persistently defy all norms, reject authority, and act only out of blind selfishness. As sociologist Lee Robins has pointed out, ASP is culturally universal: "If antisocial personality is a myth, it is a myth that is told over and over by different groups in different places and in different times, and the plot always seems to be the same."[1]

Unlike many other psychiatric disorders, including depression, schizophrenia, and attention-deficit/hyperactivity disorder

(ADHD), ASP remains under wraps from the public and only rarely are the covers pulled back far enough to afford a glimpse of the true problem. Considering its wide reach and destructive potential, ASP has an astonishingly low profile. Decades after Cleckley observed that little would be done to help individuals and society deal with psychopathy until it received full acceptance as a major health problem, we still overlook its prevalence and consequences.[2]

As a young physician fresh from medical school, I was as uninformed about ASP as anyone, at first overlooking the problem, then idealistically assuming that psychiatry could remedy it. Experience with men like Tom—my first antisocial patient (Chapter 1)—taught me that the disorder has a profound impact on the lives it touches. Years later, my belief that mental health care can help antisocials is tempered by the knowledge that its success ultimately relies on their willingness to change. Perhaps the greatest error of mental health professionals has been to ignore ASP or to mistake it for something else.

Part of the problem is the complex and disturbing nature of personality disorders themselves. Antisocial personality disorder can be understood in the crudest terms as a character flaw since at its core is a poor capacity to make moral judgments. But, as such, it raises the questions of where character comes from and how it motivates behavior. To what degree are character and personality traits inborn? If a predisposition for bad behavior exists at birth, what environmental triggers determine its emergence? Can teaching sound moral sense supplant hereditary influences? If inborn personality structures shape our actions, what happens to the concept of free will? Some implications of these questions are beyond the scope of psychiatry, but the field continues to explore fundamental issues of causation, natural history, and treatment. We may never solve the riddles of ASP but, with continued work, we should be able to make life easier for those whom it affects.

THE MYTHS

Misconceptions that circulate around ASP contribute to a collective ignorance of the disorder. Like all myths, they have a tendency to grow further from the truth with each telling and to take on lives of their own. Many are as old as the first reports of the disorder and reflect a deep discomfort with the notion that mental illness might be invoked to forgive individuals who commit terrible acts. To some people, the notion of ASP threatens to medicalize immoral behavior and excuse it from judgment. Others regard mental illnesses as less legitimate than physical ailments and their diagnosis as unreliable as the psychiatrists and psychologists who make them. Addressing these myths is part of the challenge of confronting ASP.

Antisocial personality disorder doesn't exist. Antisocial behavior clearly occurs everywhere and always. Descriptions of individuals who consistently exhibit such behavior have been written since the beginning of psychiatry nearly two centuries ago, slowly evolving into the modern notion of ASP. By carefully charting its characteristic course and outcome and by confirming its genetic roots, researchers over the past 60 years have established that ASP is a scientifically valid diagnosis. Neuroscientists are just beginning to unravel its biochemical and physiological underpinnings using state-of-the-art tools. As with many other mental and physical illnesses, scientific questions and challenges continue to surround ASP, but its history, nature, and impact offer convincing evidence of its existence. To ignore the reality of ASP is to ignore the real lives of troubled individuals whose actions and attitudes set them apart from the norm.

Antisocial personality disorder is an excuse for bad behavior. Critics of psychiatry and psychology argue that the proliferation of syndromes and disorders in official classification systems like the American Psychiatric Association's *Diagnostic and Statistical Manual of Mental Disorders* (*DSM*) threatens the notion of personal responsibility. They fear that the medicalization of bad behavior promotes the view that individuals are slaves to mental and biological processes and therefore lack control over what they do. Although some antisocials—and their attorneys—may attempt to use ASP as an excuse, psychiatrists see the disorder differently. Antisocial personality disorder describes a pattern of behaviors, choices, and feelings, but it does not mean that people with the disorder are unable to chart their own paths through life. Unlike some other mental disorders, ASP does not entail a break with reality. Antisocials know full well what is going on around them. They know the difference between right and wrong but may simply be unconcerned with it. Their actions are deliberate and focused on their self-centered goals. They are responsible for their own behavior and should be held accountable.

People with ASP are evil. Indeed, much antisocial behavior can be described as evil when judged by conventional standards of morality. But psychiatrists are not concerned with summing up an individual's moral character with a broad term like *evil*; we prefer to leave that to philosophers and theologians. Many antisocials probably qualify as evil in some people's eyes, and it is tempting to attribute their behavior to a spiritual defect. Yet antisocials are in full command of their faculties and are no more mired in a religious crisis or possessed by demons than they are legally insane. Scientific inquiry into ASP might someday trace notions of evil to biology, locating abnormalities in brain function that hinder the ability to internalize moral codes. Although such discoveries would not excuse evil, they may add another layer of complexity to discussions of morality.

"Antisocial" is another term for "criminal." There is considerable overlap between ASP and criminality, but the two are not the same. A *criminal* is someone who commits illegal acts. Antisocial personality disorder is a broad behavioral syndrome of which crime is only one aspect. Not all criminals experience the wide range of problems found among antisocials, including troubles with marriage, domestic

life, occupation, military service, education, uncontrolled aggression, and alcoholism or drug abuse. Although crime is often a significant component of ASP—and although many of the most hardened criminals are antisocial—it is hardly the only, or even the most important, symptom of the disorder. Some antisocials commit few or no crimes (or at least don't get caught), and those who stop breaking the law may continue to show other behavioral problems.

People with ASP never improve. Although many antisocials face bleak futures, the disorder has a range of outcomes and may be less severe in some cases than in others. It is wrong to assume that ASP will never get better. Although the symptoms may linger in some form throughout a patient's life, antisocial behaviors often become less frequent and severe over time. Some antisocials improve to the point at which they seem to have overcome the disorder and may no longer meet its diagnostic criteria. Nonetheless, it is clear that many different factors influence improvement and remission, including variations in the disorder itself, the influence of family and friends, and treatment for ASP and coexisting disorders.

The outlook for ASP is hopeless because there are no effective treatments. Many experts have voiced grim opinions about the treatability of ASP, but remarkable advances in the treatment of other mental disorders raise glimmers of hope. Cognitive behavioral therapy is being studied as a means to combat personality disorders. Although it remains to be seen whether this approach is the answer for antisocials, it may help some patients control their behavior. Furthermore, progress in treating illnesses like depression and ADHD with medication can provide some antisocials with relief from coexisting mental health problems, as can alcohol and drug rehabilitation. Future research may lead to drugs that specifically target ASP and its various symptoms. Finally, family therapy and marriage counseling can help rebuild bonds broken by antisocials, thus providing necessary support for overcoming the disorder.

TAKING ACTION

Armed with current knowledge of ASP, we must begin to recognize and confront the problems caused by the disorder wherever they appear. Antisocials will continue to wreak havoc in many ways and in all sorts of families and communities, and it is time we acknowledged the misery that stems from this disorder. Crime, domestic abuse, and other problems that rouse contemporary concern are often linked to ASP. Violence and serious behavioral problems among young people also are, in many cases, attributable to the disorder, which strikes early and destroys the lives of its victims—both those who have it and those around them. Antisocial personality disorder causes suffering among the children of antisocials, whether or not they go on to develop the disorder themselves. Its financial costs to society—lost productivity, law enforcement, incarceration, medical care—are enormous, but the human costs are still larger and much more devastating.

Understanding the scope of the disorder and coming to grips with it will require time and money. Government agencies and private foundations need to earmark funds for studies of ASP and its many facets, especially crime and violence. Research on the causes and prevention of violence is politically unpopular in many camps—from those who fear the racial implications of studies on violence and genetics to others concerned that public health approaches to the problem will threaten gun ownership rights. Still more obstacles to research on ASP come from those who believe the myths described above. "Get-tough" attitudes toward crime, harsh attitudes toward sentencing, and other popular ideas may be summoned against any project that gives the impression of excusing or coddling criminal behavior. Psychiatrists and other experts must continue to spread information about ASP to quell misconceptions.

Mental health professionals must overcome their own resistance to working with antisocials if they are to develop new treatments and prevention strategies. Such work takes dedication, perseverance, and a deep understanding of the disorder, and training in the mental health professions should address the challenges and demands of treating antisocials. The short-term rewards may be less satisfying than those to be gained from treating other types of patients, but all of us working to treat mental illnesses must remain focused on long-term goals as well. Our success in preventing and treating ASP will have a broad impact that ripples through society, helping to reduce spousal abuse, family violence, and criminal behavior.

Research priorities should include wide-ranging projects to explore the origins of ASP and search for methods to change its course. Geneticists must continue to investigate the mechanisms behind the hereditary transmission of the disorder, locating genes that might predispose individuals to ASP and determining how these genes function at the molecular level. Neuroscientists should work to pinpoint brain regions or networks linked to antisocial behavior, while identifying the biochemical and physiological pathways that influence its expression. A full range of treatments, including drugs and psychotherapy, need to be developed, tested, and refined. Last, we must focus attention on the group at highest risk of developing ASP—namely, children with a conduct disorder. Improved understanding of their home life and social environment may lead to more effective interventions to prevent ASP from developing.

The implications of ASP for law enforcement and criminal justice must be taken seriously. By improving records and communication, we could more easily spot patterns of crime, especially in young offenders. Concern for privacy and procedure must be balanced with efforts to derail criminal careers before they fully develop. When lawyers for antisocial defendants use the diagnosis to help clients evade responsibility, juries and judges should view their efforts with skepticism. When antisocial criminals are identified, the criminal justice system must consider the nature of the disorder in sentencing—understanding, for example, that ASP often diminishes with age, making older criminals less menacing than they were in their younger years. Because conventional prison rehabilitation programs have uncertain results, efforts to develop effective therapeutic programs for antisocials should be explored if we are to reduce the threat they pose when released back onto the streets. As we come to recognize the impact of personality disorders on crime, we should ensure that preventive detention in hospitals does not replace prison terms. Prisons are the best place for dangerous offenders, although simply putting antisocials behind bars will do little to alleviate the causes of their problems.

Antisocials should be encouraged to seek help, as should those who live with them. Antisocial personality disorder erodes family bonds, holds spouses and partners captive in relationships built on intimidation, and condemns children to years of neglect and abuse. It is a problem no one should have to live with, but many do. Resources must be available for all involved, from programs for victims of abuse to ASP treatment options from qualified mental health professionals.

The problem of individuals who proceed through life outside all manner of social regulation has long been with us under many names: *manie sans délire, moral insanity, psychopathy, sociopathic personality, ASP.* Whatever we call it, the condition remains all around us, largely unrecognized for what it is. It is time for that to change. The men I have described throughout these pages could be neighbors, family members, or friends whose behavior swings from simply frustrating to deeply disturbing. Directly or indirectly, nearly all of us are affected by ASP at some point. We know antisocials, are victims of their misdeeds, fear them, or even grapple with the disorder ourselves. Antisocial personality disorder explains a longstanding observation about the human condition: Some of us seem to be born bad. Now more than ever, psychiatry and society have the means to explore why bad boys become bad men, how we can stop them, and how to mend the damage they cause. Progress will continue if we begin to see this phenomenon more clearly and commit ourselves to doing something about it. If nothing else, confronting ASP will teach us something more about what it means to be part of a family, a community, and a culture, bound as we are by certain rules, expectations, and our own sense of conscience. In seeing what antisocials lack, we may be all the more grateful for what we have.

NOTES

Introduction

1. Donald Goodwin and Samuel Guze, *Psychiatric Diagnosis*, 4th ed. (New York: Oxford University Press, 1989), 240.
2. Lack of remorse was found in 51% of antisocials assessed in a large national survey (NESARC). See Risë B. Goldstein, Bridget F. Grant, Boji Huang, et al., "Lack of remorse in antisocial personality disorder: sociodemographic correlates, symptomatic presentation, and comorbidity with Axis I and Axis II disorders in the National Epidemiologic Survey on Alcohol and Related Conditions," *Comprehensive Psychiatry* 47 (2006): 289–297.
3. Ann Rule, *The Stranger Beside Me* (New York: Penguin Books, 1989), 397.

1. A Lurking Threat

1. The NESARC study is the latest of several large-scale epidemiologic surveys in the United States that show the high rate of ASP in the general population. This and other major studies have used standardized diagnostic interviews and probability sampling procedures that are state-of-the-art. The NESARC was preceded by the National Comorbidity Study-Replication, which found an overall rate for ASP of 3.5%, whereas the older ECA study reported a figure of 2.5%. Information on lifetime prevalence of psychiatric disorders appears in the following articles: William M. Compton, Kevin P. Conway, Frederick S. Stinson, et al., "Prevalence, correlates, and comorbidity of DSM-IV antisocial personality syndromes and alcohol and specific drug use disorders in the United States: results from the National Epidemiologic Survey on Alcohol and Related Conditions," *Journal of Clinical Psychiatry* 66 (2005):677–685; Deborah S. Hasin, Renee D. Goodwin, Frederick S. Stinson, et al., "Epidemiology of major depression—results from the National Epidemiologic Survey on Alcoholism and Related Conditions," *Archives of General Psychiatry* 62 (2005):1097–1106;

Bridget F. Grant, Deborah S. Hasin, Frederick S. Stinson, et al., "The epidemiology of DSM-IV panic disorder and agoraphobia in the United States: results from the National Epidemiologic Survey on Alcohol and Related Conditions," *Journal of Clinical Psychiatry* 67 (2006): 363–374; Ronald C. Kessler, Patricia Berglund, Olga Demler, et al., "Lifetime prevalence and age-of-onset distributions of DSM-IV disorders in the National Comorbidity Study Replication," *Archives of General Psychiatry* 62 (2005): 593–602; Lee N. Robins, John E. Helzer, Myrna M. Weissman, et al., "Lifetime prevalence of specific psychiatric disorders in three sites," *Archives of General Psychiatry* 41 (1984): 949–958; and Ronald C. Kessler, Lenard Adler, and Russell Barkley, et al., "The prevalence and correlates of adult ADHD in the United States: results from the National Comorbidity Survey Replication," *American Journal of Psychiatry* 163 (2006):716–723.

2. Donald W. Black, Connie H. Baumgard, and Sue E. Bell, "A 16- to 45-year follow-up of 71 males with antisocial personality disorder," *Comprehensive Psychiatry* 36 (1995): 130–140.

3. This figure comes from the U.S. Bureau of Justice Statistics, which lists 2,266,800 persons as incarcerated in jails and prisons in 2010. Accessed February 29, 2012, at http://bjs.ojp.usdoj.gov.

4. The figure is calculated by taking into account the estimated 2011 U.S. population (311 million). Seventy-six percent of the population is over 18 years, a requirement for ASP, which yields an at-risk population of 236 million. With an ASP prevalence of 3.6%, about 8.5 million people are antisocial (www.census.gov).

5. William Bennett, *The Book of Virtues: A Treasury of Great Moral Stories* (New York: Simon & Schuster, 1993).

6. Alan Dershowitz, *The Abuse Excuse and Other Copouts, Sob Stories and Evasions of Responsibility* (New York: Little, Brown, 1994).

7. An example of anticrime rhetoric, politics, and the law is the 1994 federal crime bill. Passed by a bare majority in both houses of Congress, the bill called for an expansion in the number of police officers in major cities, mandated tougher sentencing guidelines, and expanded the number of federal crimes punishable by death. Whether such bills have any impact on the crime rate is questionable. See "Experts Doubt Effectiveness of Crime Bill," *New York Times*, September 14, 1994.

8. O. J.'s life and courtroom battles are reported in Theresa Carpenter's "The man behind the mask," *Esquire*, November 1994, 84–100; and in Dominick Dunne's "L.A. in the Age of O. J.," *Vanity Fair*, February 1995, 46–56; for information about his 2008 trial, see "Nevada: Simpson Appeals," *New York Times*, October 11, 2008.

9. See Lisa Pulitzer and Cole Thompson, *Portrait of a Monster: Joran van der Sloot, a Murder in Peru, and the Natalee Holloway Mystery* (New York: St. Martin's Press, 2011).

10. "Portrait of a Real Hobo—Footloose, Fighting, Sometimes Bitter," *Des Moines Register*, September 24, 1990.

11. Antisocial behavior is a staple in the book trade. Some books in my home library that center on antisocial behavior and personalities include:

    And the Sea Will Tell, Vincent Bugliosi and Bruce B. Henderson (New York: W. W. Norton, 1991)

    Bad Guys, Mark Baker (New York: Dell, 1997)

    Blind Eye—How the Medical Establishment Let a Doctor Get Away with Murder, James B. Stewart (New York: Simon & Schuster, 1999)

    Brothers in Blood, Clark Howard (New York: St. Martin's Press, 1983)

    Clockers, Richard Price (New York: Houghton Mifflin, 1992)

    Columbine, Dave Cullen (New York: Twelve, 2009)

    Echoes in the Darkness, Joseph Wambaugh (New York: Perigord, 1987)

    First Sins of Ross Michael Carlson, Michael Weissberg (New York: Dell, 1992)

    Girl Wanted: The Chase for Sarah Pender, Steve Miller (New York, Berkley Prime, 2011)

    Most Evil: Avenger, Zodiac, and Further Serial Murders of Dr. George Hill Hodel, Steve Hodel (New York: Dutton, 2009)

    Nutcracker, Shana Alexander (New York: Doubleday, 1985)

    Richie, Thomas Thompson (New York: E. P. Dutton, 1981)

    Savage, Robert Scott (New York: Pinnacle, 2002)

    Sex Crimes, Alice Vachss (New York: Henry Holt, 1993)

    Shadow of Cain, Vincent Bugliosi and Ken Horwitz (New York: W. W. Norton, 1981)

    "Son": A Psychopath and His Victims, Jack Olsen (New York: Atheneum, 1983)

    The Dark Son, Denise Lang (New York: Avon Books, 1995)

    The Misbegotten Son, Jack Olsen (New York: Delacorte Press, 1993)

    To Hear and Obey, Lawrence Taylor (New York: William Morrow, 1992)

    When a Child Kills, Paul Mones (New York: Pocket Books, 1991)

    Without Pity, Ann Rule (New York: Pocket Books, 2003).

12. Carole Lieberman and Lisa Collier, *Bad Boys: Why We Love Them, How to Live with Them, and When to Leave Them* (New York: Dutton, 1997).

13. Truman Capote, *In Cold Blood: A True Account of Multiple Murder and Its Consequences* (New York: New American Library, 1965).

14. Mikal Gilmore, *Shot in the Heart* (New York: Doubleday, 1994). Gilmore presents recollections of his grossly dysfunctional family, most of whom are antisocial to some extent. The book is funny, sad, poignant, disturbing, and utterly fascinating.

15. The prevalence of ASP has been studied in countries around the globe and these studies confirm not only its universality, but also that criteria used to define the disorder in the United States are relevant elsewhere. See Char-Nie Chen, Jesse Wong, Nancy Lee, et al., "The Shatin community mental health survey in Hong Kong: II. Major findings," *Archives of General Psychiatry* 50

(1993): 125–133; J. Elizabeth Wells, John A. Bushnell, Andrew R. Hornblow, et al., "Christchurch Psychiatric Epidemiology Study: Part I. Methodology and lifetime prevalence for specific psychiatric disorders," *Australia and New Zealand Journal of Psychiatry* 23 (1989): 315–326; Chung Kyoon Lee, Young Sook Kwak, Joe Yamamoto, et al., "Psychiatric epidemiology in Korea: Part I. Gender and age differences in Seoul," *Journal of Nervous and Mental Disease* 178 (1990): 242–252. A study in Taiwan found much lower rates of ASP. See Wilson M. Compton, John E. Helzer, Hai-Gwo Hwu, et al., "New methods in cross-cultural psychiatry: psychiatric illness in Taiwan and the United States," *American Journal of Psychiatry* 148 (1994): 1697–1704. The investigators suggest that there is either a true difference in the prevalence of ASP or that the types of antisocial acts required for the diagnosis may be infrequent in relatively rigid societies.

16. Lee N. Robins, "The Epidemiology of Antisocial Personality Disorder," in *Psychiatry*, Volume 3, Chapter 19, eds. Robert O. Michels and Jesse O. Cavenar (Philadelphia: J. B. Lippincott, 1987), 1–14; see also Gerald Nestadt, Alan J. Romanoski, Jack F. Samuels, et al., "The relationship between personality and DSM-III axis I disorders in the population: results from an epidemiologic survey," *American Journal of Psychiatry* 149 (1992): 1228–1233.

17. See Landy F. Sparr, "Personality disorders and criminal law: an international perspective," *Journal of the American Academy of Psychiatry and the Law* 37 (2009): 168–181.

18. Of the thousands of projects funded by National Institutes of Health (NIH), only 79 projects come up when "antisocial personality" is entered as a topic into the NIH RePORTER website, meaning that this has been suggested as a "key word" by the researchers. Only two projects have "antisocial" in the title, four list "conduct," and five list "psychopathy" or "psychopath" (http://projectreporter.nih.gov/reporter.cmf, accessed March 2, 2012).

19. George Winokur, MD, had directed the Iowa 500 studies—considered classics in the psychiatric research—in which the natural course of depression, mania, and schizophrenia were determined. See John Clancy, Ming-Tso Tsuang, Barbara Norton, and George Winokur, "The Iowa 500: A comprehensive study of mania, depression, and schizophrenia," *Journal of the Iowa Medical Society* 64 (1974): 394–398; and Ming-Tso Tsuang, Robert F. Woolson, and Jerome A. Fleming, "Long-term outcome of major psychoses: I. Schizophrenia and affective disorders compared with psychiatrically symptom-free surgical conditions," *Archives of General Psychiatry* 36 (1979): 1295–1301.

20. My study of 71 antisocial men is summarized in four articles. See Donald W. Black, Connie H. Baumgard, and Sue E. Bell, "A 16- to 45-year follow-up of 71 males with antisocial personality disorder," *Comprehensive Psychiatry* 36 (1995): 130–140; Donald W. Black, Connie H. Baumgard, and Sue E. Bell, "The long-term outcome of antisocial personality disorder compared with depression, schizophrenia, and surgical conditions," *Bulletin of the American*

Academy of Psychiatry and the Law 23 (1995): 43–51; Donald W. Black, Connie H. Baumgard, Sue E. Bell, and Chi Kao, "Death rates in 71 men with antisocial personality disorder: a comparison with general population mortality," *Psychosomatics* 37 (1996): 131–136; and Donald W. Black, Patrick O. Monahan, Connie H. Baumgard, and Sue E. Bell, "Predictors of long-term outcome in antisocial personality disorder," *Annals of Clinical Psychiatry* 9 (1997): 211–217.

2. Searching for Answers

1. See Ephraim Karsh and Inari Rautsi, *Saddam Hussein: A Political Biography* (New York: Brassey's, 1991), esp. 267–268.
2. American Psychiatric Association, *Diagnostic and Statistical Manual of Mental Disorders*, 4th ed. (Washington, D.C.: American Psychiatric Press, 1994), 629.
3. The case is cited in George Winokur and Raymond Crowe, "Personality Disorders," in *Comprehensive Textbook of Psychiatry*, Volume II, eds. Arthur M. Freedman, Harold I. Kaplan, and Benjamin J. Sadock (Baltimore: Williams & Wilkins, 1975), 1287.
4. Rush's quotation appears in Michael Craft, "The Meanings of the Term Psychopath," in *Psychopathic Disorders*, ed. Michael Craft (New York: Pergamon Press, 1966), 15.
5. Prichard is quoted in Donald Goodwin and Samuel Guze, *Psychiatric Diagnosis*, 4th ed. (New York: Oxford University Press, 1989), 240.
6. David Henderson, *Psychopathic States* (New York: W. W. Norton, 1939).
7. Hervey Cleckley, *The Mask of Sanity: An Attempt to Clarify Some Issues About the So-Called Psychopathic Personality*, 5th ed. (St. Louis: C. V. Mosby, 1976). This book has been very influential to generations of psychiatrists and is required reading in many psychiatry training programs.
8. Ibid., 33.
9. Ibid.
10. American Psychiatric Association, *Diagnostic and Statistical Manual of Mental Disorders* (Washington, D.C.: American Psychiatric Association, 1952).
11. American Psychiatric Association, *Diagnostic and Statistical Manual of Mental Disorders*, 2nd ed. (Washington, D.C.: American Psychiatric Association, 1968).
12. American Psychiatric Association, *Diagnostic and Statistical Manual of Mental Disorders*, 3rd ed. (Washington, D.C.: American Psychiatric Press, 1980).
13. Lee N. Robins, *Deviant Children Grown Up* (Baltimore: Williams & Wilkins, 1966).
14. The process of developing the DSM-III criteria is described by Martyn Pickersgill in "Standardising antisocial personality disorder: the social shaping of psychiatric technology," *Sociology of Health & Illness* (2011). Published online October 21, 2011, DOI: 10.1111/j.1467-9566.2011.01404.x.

15. American Psychiatric Association, *Diagnostic and Statistical Manual of Mental Disorders*, 3rd ed. Revised (Washington, D.C.: American Psychiatric Association, 1987); American Psychiatric Association, *Diagnostic and Statistical Manual of Mental Disorders*, 4th ed. (Washington, D.C.: American Psychiatric Association, 1994); American Psychiatric Association, *Diagnostic and Statistical Manual of Mental Disorders*, 4th ed. Text Revision (Washington, D.C.: American Psychiatric Association, 2000). For information on *DSM-5*, currently in development, visit: http://www.dsm5.org.

16. Robert D. Hare, *Without Conscience—The Disturbing World of the Psychopaths Among Us* (New York: Pocket Books, 1993).

17. See Robert D. Hare, "Diagnosis of antisocial personality disorder in two prison populations," *American Journal of Psychiatry* 140 (1983): 887–890; Mark D. Cunningham, Thomas J. Reidy, "Antisocial personality disorder and psychopathy: diagnostic dilemmas in classifying patterns of antisocial behavior in sentence evaluations," *Behavioral Science and the Law* 18 (1998): 333–351; and Jeremy Coid and Simone Ullrich, "Antisocial personality disorder is on a continuum with psychopathy," *Comprehensive Psychiatry* 51 (2010): 426–433.

18. See Coid and Ullrich (2010).

19. Megan J. Rutherford, Arthur I. Alterman, John S. Cacciola, and Edward Snider, "Gender differences in diagnosing antisocial personality in methadone patients," *American Journal of Psychiatry* 152 (1995): 1309–1316.

20. For information on ASP and poverty, see Lee N. Robins, "Epidemiology of antisocial personality disorder," in *Psychiatry*, Volume 3, Chapter 19, eds. Robert O. Michels and Jesse O. Cavenar (Philadelphia: J. B. Lippincott, 1987), 1–14. On homelessness and ASP, see Carol North, Elizabeth M. Smith, and Edward L. Spitznagel, "Is antisocial personality a valid diagnosis in the homeless?" *American Journal of Psychiatry* 150 (1993): 578–583.

21. See Samuel Guze, *Criminality and Psychiatric Disorders* (New York: Oxford University Press, 1976). In a follow-up study of 223 felons, Guze reported that 79% met criteria for ASP at intake into the study, and 60% met criteria eight or nine years later; 81% met criteria for ASP at either one of the interviews. In a study of 66 female felons, 65% were judged to have ASP. A lower figure (39%) is used by Robert Hare. See Robert D. Hare, "Diagnosis of antisocial personality disorder in two prison populations," *American Journal of Psychiatry* 140 (1983): 887–890.

22. See Donald W. Black, Tracy Gunter, Peggy Loveless, et al., "Antisocial personality disorder in incarcerated offenders: psychiatric comorbidity and quality of life," *Annals of Clinical Psychiatry* 22 (2010): 113–120.

23. Adrian Raine, *The Psychopathology of Crime* (New York: Academic Press, 1993).

24. The reported prevalence of ASP among alcoholics ranges from 16% to 49%, and the figures among heroin addicts and cocaine-dependent patients are

still higher. For a review of ASP's effect on addictive disorders, see Victor Hesselbrock, Roger Meyer, and Michie Hesselbrock, "Psychopathology and Addictive Disorders: The Specific Case of Antisocial Personality Disorder," in *Addictive States*, eds. C. P. O'Brien and J. H. Jaffe (New York: Raven Press, 1992), 179–191.

25. K. L. Barry, M. F. Fleming, L. B. Maxwell, et al., "Conduct disorder and anti-social personality in adult primary care patients," *Journal of Family Practice* 45 (1997): 151–158.

26. Lee N. Robins, John E. Helzer, Myrna M. Weissman, et al., "Lifetime prevalence of specific psychiatric disorders in three sites," *Archives of General Psychiatry* 41 (1984): 949–958. For a discussion of reasons for lower prevalence rates in older antisocials, see Bruce J. Cohen, Gerald Nestadt, Jack F. Samuels, et al., "Personality disorder in late life: a community study," *British Journal of Psychiatry* 165 (1994): 493–499.

27. Julio Arboleda-Florez and Heather L. Holley, "Antisocial burn-out: an explor-atory study," *Bulletin of the American Academy of Psychiatry and the Law* 19 (1991): 173–183.

28. African Americans and whites show a similar prevalence of ASP. In a reanaly-sis of the ECA data, Lee N. Robins reports that childhood conduct prob-lems occurred at much higher rates in African Americans than in whites but that African Americans were less likely than whites to continue these behav-iors into adult life, resulting in similar rates of ASP. See "The Epidemiology of Antisocial Personality Disorder," in *Psychiatry*, Volume 3, Chapter 19, eds. Robert O. Michels and Jesse O. Cavenar (Philadelphia: J. B. Lippincott, 1987), 4–5. For rates of ASP among Mexican Americans, see Marvin Karno, Richard L. Hough, Audrey Burham, et al., "Lifetime prevalence of specific psychiatric disorders among Mexican-Americans and non-Hispanic whites in Los Angeles," *Archives of General Psychiatry* 44 (1987): 695–701. In the more recent National Epidemiologic Survey on Alcohol and Related Conditions (NESARC), Native Americans were at increased risk for ASP, whereas Asian Americans and Hispanic respondents had *lower* risk than whites. See William M. Compton, Kevin P. Conway, Frederick S. Stinson, et al., "Prevalence, correlates, and comorbidity of DSM-IV antisocial personality syndromes and alcohol and specific drug use disorders in the United States: results from the National Epidemiologic Survey on Alcohol and Related Conditions," *Journal of Clinical Psychiatry* 66 (2005): 677–685.

3. Bad Boys to Bad Men

1. The criteria for both conduct disorder and ASP are contained in the American Psychiatric Association's *Diagnostic and Statistical Manual of Mental Disorders*,

4th ed. Text Revision (Washington, D.C.: American Psychiatric Association, 2000).

2. Charles W. Popper and Ronald J. Steingard, "Disorders Usually First Diagnosed in Infancy, Childhood, or Adolescence," in *The American Psychiatric Press Textbook of Psychiatry*, 2nd ed. (Washington, D.C.: American Psychiatric Press, 1994), 729–832.

3. "There Are No Children Here," *Time*, September 12, 1994. See also "Falling" by Adrian Nicole LeBlanc, *Esquire*, April 1995, 84–100; and "In an 11-year-old's Funeral a Grim Lesson," *New York Times*, September 8, 1994.

4. "Inside the Mind of a Child Killer," *Turning Point*, ABC Network, December 14, 1994.

5. See Hara Estroff Marano, "Big Bad Bully," *Psychology Today*, September/October 1995, 50–82.

6. See Kathryn L. Falb, Heather L. McCauley, Michele R. Decker, et al., "School bullying perpetration and other childhood risk factors as predictors of intimate partner violence perpetration," *Archives of Pediatrics and Adolescent Medicine* 165 (2011): 890–894. The connection between early childhood aggression and adult violence is amply documented. For a review of 14 studies confirming this phenomenon, see Rolf Loeber and Magda Stouthammer-Loeber, "Prediction," in *Handbook of Juvenile Delinquency*, ed. Herbert C. Quay (New York: John Wiley & Sons, 1987), 325–382.

7. See Daniel S. Hellman and Nathan Blackman, "Enuresis, firesetting, and cruelty to animals: a triad predictive of adult crime," *American Journal of Psychiatry* 122 (1966): 1431–1435.

8. See John C. Pomeroy, David Behar, and Mark A. Stewart, "Abnormal sexual behavior in prepubescent children," *British Journal of Psychiatry* 138 (1981): 119–125; see also Alayne Yates, "Children eroticized by incest," *American Journal of Psychiatry* 139 (1982): 482–485.

9. "Shabazz Youth Admits Setting the Fatal Fire," *New York Times*, July 11, 1997; "Psychologist Says Malcomb Shabazz a Firebug Since Age 3," Associated Press, July 30, 1997; and "Prosecutors Want Media Out of Shabazz Case," *Chicago Tribune*, June 25, 1997.

10. Eugene Methvin, "The Face of Evil," *National Review*, January 23, 1995, 34–44.

11. See Dave Cullen, *Columbine* (New York: Twelve, 2009).

12. Jill Smolow, "Parenting on trial: a Michigan couple is fined for a son's crimes," *Time*, May 20, 1996, 50.

13. Lee N. Robins, "The Epidemiology of Antisocial Personality," in *Psychiatry*, Volume 3, Chapter 19, eds. Robert O. Michels and Jesse O. Cavenar (Philadelphia: J. B. Lippincott, 1987), 1–14; Mark Zoccolillo, Andrew Pickles, David Quinton, and Michael Rutter cite similar figures in "The outcome of childhood conduct disorder: implications for defining adult personality disorder and conduct disorder," *Psychological Medicine* 22 (1992): 971–986. They report that 40% of boys and 35% of girls with conduct

disorder developed adult ASP. More than two-thirds had "pervasive and persistent social malfunction."

14. Lee N. Robins, *Deviant Children Grown Up* (Baltimore: Williams & Wilkins, 1966), 111.

15. "Anti-violence Activists Wonder Why Proctor Wasn't in Prison," *Des Moines Register*, December 5, 1995.

16. See Joshua Quittner, "Kevin Mitnik's Digital Obsession," *Time*, February 27, 1995, 45.

17. "Yale Says Impostor Is Studying in the Ivy," *New York Times*, April 4, 1995.

18. Courtney Leatherman, "Numerous academics have been duped by a scam using names of prominent scholars," *Chronicle of Higher Education*, May 23, 1997.

19. Mikal Gilmore, *Shot in the Heart* (New York: Doubleday, 1994), 79–80.

20. "Portrait of a Real Hobo—Footloose, Fighting, Sometimes Bitter," *Des Moines Register*, September 25, 1990.

21. For information on the psychiatric status of the homeless, see Carol S. North, Elizabeth M. Smith, and Edward L. Spitznagel, "Is antisocial personality a valid diagnosis among the homeless?" *American Journal of Psychiatry* 150 (1993): 578–583; and Paul Koegel, Audrey Burnam, and Roger K. Farr, "The prevalence of specific psychiatric disorders among homeless individuals in the inner city of Los Angeles," *Archives of General Psychiatry* 45 (1988): 1085–1092.

22. The trouble-prone boxer's early years are explored by Pete Hamilton in "The education of Mike Tyson," *Esquire*, March 1994, 99–106. For news on Tyson's recent exploits, visit http://en.wikipedia.org/wiki/Mike_Tyson (accessed March 2, 2012).

23. In *Deviant Children Grown Up*, Robins showed that 38% of non-antisocial controls had never been injured accidentally, compared with 16% of antisocials (93). The relationship between ASP and accidental injury also is discussed by Robert A. Woodruff, Samuel B. Guze, and Paula J. Clayton in "The medical and psychiatric implications of antisocial personality (sociopathy)," *Diseases of the Nervous System* 32 (1971): 712–714.

24. See Donald W. Black, Connie Baumgard, Sue E. Bell, and Chi Kao, "Death rates in 71 men with antisocial personality disorder: a comparison with general population mortality," *Psychosomatics* 37 (1996): 131–136. Robins reported in *Deviant Children Grown Up* that antisocials had a higher overall death rate from "natural causes, war, and accidents" (91).

25. The problem of HIV infection in ASP is discussed by Robert K. Brooner, Lawrence Greenfield, Chester W. Schmidt, and George E. Bigelow in "Antisocial personality disorder and HIV infection among intravenous drug abusers," *American Journal of Psychiatry* 150 (1993): 53–58. The authors compared drug abusers with and without ASP. Eighteen percent of drug abusers with ASP were HIV positive compared with 8% of abusers without ASP. The authors concluded that the diagnosis of ASP was associated with a significantly

higher odds ratio of HIV infection independent of ethnicity, gender, and treatment status.

26. Robins, *Deviant Children Grown Up*, 95–101.

27. Samuel B. Guze, *Criminality and Psychiatric Disorders* (New York: Oxford University Press, 1976).

28. Lee N. Robins and R. G. Lewis portray antisocials as incompetent parents in "The role of the antisocial family in school completion and delinquency," *Sociology Quarterly* 7 (1966): 500–514; see also Yuriko Egami, Daniel E. Ford, Shelly F. Greenfield, and Rosa M. Crum, "Psychiatric profile and sociodemographic characteristics of adults who report physically abusing or neglecting children," *American Journal of Psychiatry* 153 (1996): 921–928.

29. "Uncertain Future, on Their Own, Awaits," *New York Times*, March 16, 1997.

30. For a discussion of disturbed social relationships in antisocials, see Robins, *Deviant Children Grown Up*, 115–118.

31. See Risë B. Goldstein, Sally I. Powers, Jane McCusker, et al., "Lack of remorse in antisocial personality disorder among drug abusers in residential treatment," *Journal of Personality Disorders* 10 (1996): 321–334; and Risë B. Goldstein, Bridget F. Grant, Boji Huang, et al., "Lack of remorse in antisocial personality disorder: Sociodemographic correlates, symptomatic presentation, and comorbidity with Axis I and Axis II disorders in the National Epidemiologic Survey on Alcohol and Related Conditions," *Comprehensive Psychiatry* 47 (2006): 289–297.

32. Tim Cahill and Russ Ewing, *Buried Dreams: Inside the Mind of a Serial Killer* (New York: Bantam Books, 1986), 371.

33. "Repeat Sex Offender Says He Is the Victim," *Cedar Rapids Gazette*, April 14, 1997.

34. Jack Henry Abbott, *In the Belly of the Beast* (New York: Vintage Books, 1981), xi–xii. For information about Abbott's life post prison, see http://en.wikipedia. org/wiki/jack_abbott (accessed April 3, 2012).

35. Robins, *Deviant Children Grown Up*, 49.

36. Ibid., 42–73.

37. See Lee N. Robins, "The Epidemiology of Antisocial Personality," in *Psychiatry*, Volume 3, Chapter 19, eds. Robert O. Michels and Jesse O. Cavenar (Philadelphia: J. B. Lippincott, 1987); and Risë B. Goldstein, Sally I. Powers, Jane McCusker, et al., "Gender differences in manifestations of antisocial personality disorder among residential drug abuse treatment clients," *Drug and Alcohol Dependence* 41 (1996): 35–45.

38. As an example of gender differences in incarcerated offenders, see Tracy Gunter, Gloria Wenman, Bruce Sieleni, et al., "Frequency of mental health and addictive disorders among 320 men and women entering the Iowa prison system," *Journal of the American Academy of Psychiatry and the Law* 36 (2008): 27–34.

39. Kent Walker, *Son of a Grifter* (New York: Avon Books, 2001). Also see David Rhode, "Mother and Son Guilty of Killing a Socialite Who Vanished in '98," *New York Times*, May 19, 2000; and "Life Terms for Pair," *New York Times*, March 22, 2005.

40. See Goldstein, Powers, and McCuster, 1996.

41. See Wendy S. Slutske, "The genetics of antisocial behavior," *Current Psychiatry Reports* 3 (2001): 158–162.

42. Donald W. Black, Tracy Gunter, Peggy Loveless, et al., "Antisocial personality disorder in incarcerated offenders: psychiatric comorbidity and quality of life," *Annals of Clinical Psychiatry* 22 (2010): 113–120.

4. Naming the Problem

1. Treatment-seeking behavior in antisocials surveyed in the ECA is described by Sam Shapiro, Elizabeth A. Skinner, Larry G. Kessler, et al., in "Utilization of health and mental health services," *Archives of General Psychiatry* 14 (1984): 971–978; and by Darrel A. Regier, William E. Narrow, Donald S. Rae, et al., in "The de facto U.S. mental and addictive disorders service system," *Archives of General Psychiatry* 50 (1993): 85–94. For recent data from the United Kingdom, see Simone Ullrich and Jeremy Coid, "Antisocial personality disorder: co-morbid Axis I mental disorders and health service utilization among a national household population," *Personality and Mental Health* 3 (2009): 151–164.

2. Hervey Cleckley, *The Mask of Sanity: An Attempt to Clarify Some Issues About the So-Called Psychopathic Personality*, 5th ed. (St. Louis: C. V. Mosby, 1976), 383.

3. For a discussion of the psychiatric assessment, see "Interviewing and Assessment," by Donald W. Black and Nancy C. Andreasen, in the *Introductory Textbook of Psychiatry*, 5th ed. (Washington, D.C.: American Psychiatric Publishing, Inc. 2011), 41–89. In this chapter, my colleague and I provide a detailed description of the methods used in assessing psychiatric patients.

4. Nancy C. Andreasen, John Rice, Jean Endicott, et al., "The family history approach to diagnosis: how useful is it?" *Archives of General Psychiatry* 43 (1986): 421–429.

5. Patricia Green, Diane Watts, Sabrina Poole, and Vasant Dhopesh, "Why patients sign out against medical advice (AMA): factors motivating patients to sign out AMA," *American Journal of Drug and Alcohol Abuse* 30 (2004): 489–493.

6. See Marshall D. Schechter, "Adoption," in *Comprehensive Textbook of Psychiatry*, 5th ed., eds. Harold I. Kaplan and Benjamin J. Sadock (Baltimore: Williams & Wilkins, 1989), 1958–1962. Although 1% to 2% of the general population is adopted, the figure among antisocials is about 15%. Adoptees are also more

likely to have behavior problems than are nonadoptees. An estimated 10% to 15% of patients seen by child psychiatrists are adoptees.

7. Daniel S. Hellman and Nathan Blackman, "Enuresis, firesetting, and cruelty to animals: a triad predictive of adult crime," *American Journal of Psychiatry* 122 (1966): 1431–1435; see also Sheldon Glueck and Eleanor Glueck, *Unraveling Juvenile Delinquency* (New York: The Commonwealth Fund, 1960), 171. They report that 28% of delinquent youth were bedwetters compared to 15% of non-delinquent youth.

8. The MMPI was developed in the 1940s, and its terminology reflects concepts and words in use at the time. A typical MMPI profile for antisocials shows peaks on Scale 4 (psychopathic deviance) and Scale 9 (hypomania), referred to as the *4–9 profile*. See W. G. Dahlstrom, G. S. Welsh, and L. E. Dahlstrom, *An MMPI Handbook* (Minneapolis: University of Minnesota Press, 1972).

9. Stephen D. Hart, Phillip R. Kropp, and Robert. D. Hare, "Performance of male psychopaths following conditional release from prison," *Journal of Consulting and Clinical Psychology* 56 (1988): 227–232. In a study of 231 male prison inmates categorized as psychopaths (Psychopathy Checklist score of ≥34) or nonpsychopaths (score of ≤24), 65% of the psychopaths violated their release conditions compared with 24% of the nonpsychopaths. A briefer screening version of the PCL-R is available.

10. For information on the Rorschach and its use in antisocials and psychopaths, see J. Reid Meloy and Carl B. Gacano, "The Internal World of the Psychopath," *Psychopathy: Antisocial, Criminal, and Violent Behavior*, eds. Theodore Millon, Erik Simonsen, Morten Birket-Smith, and Roger D. Davis (New York: Guilford, 2003), 95–109.

11. For an interesting discussion of intelligence and antisocial behavior, see Adrian Raine, *The Psychopathology of Crime* (New York: Academic Press, 1993), 232–235.

12. Stanton E. Samenow, *Inside the Criminal Mind* (New York: Times Books, 1984), 8.

13. Many questionnaires and structured interviews can be used to assess for the presence of ASP and other personality disorders. A partial list includes the Structured Interview for DSM-IV Personality, the Personality Diagnostic Questionnaire-IV, the Structured Clinical Interview for DSM-IV Personality Disorders, and the International Personality Disorder Examination.

14. Betty A. Walker and Eugene Ziskind found that 48% of 62 antisocials were nail biters compared with 24% of 62 controls. See "Relationship of nailbiting to sociopathy," *Journal of Nervous and Mental Disease* 164 (1977): 64–65.

15. Tattoos have long been associated with ASP and are discussed by Armando Favazza in *Bodies Under Siege: Self-Mutilation in Culture and Psychiatry* (Baltimore: Johns Hopkins University Press, 1987); by Gustave Newman in "The implications of tattooing in prisoners," *Journal of Clinical Psychiatry* 43

(1982): 231–234; and by William Cardasis, Alissa Huth-Bocks, and Kenneth R. Silk, in "Tattoos and antisocial personality disorder," *Personality and Mental Health* 2 (2008): 171–182. In 36 forensic psychiatric inpatients, tattoos were significantly related to an ASP diagnosis. Men with ASP had a significantly greater number of tattoos and a greater percentage of their body surface tattooed than did those without ASP.

5. Divergent Paths

1. Lee N. Robins, "Sturdy childhood predictors of adult antisocial behavior: replications from longitudinal studies," *Psychological Medicine* 8 (1978): 611. Although most antisocial children do not become antisocial adults, Robins shows that adult ASP is virtually always associated with childhood conduct disorder. She also found that adult antisocial behavior was better predicted by childhood behavior than by any other single variable.
2. The Gluecks published a number of books on their studies of delinquent children in 1940s and 1950s Boston, including *Unraveling Juvenile Delinquency* (Cambridge: Harvard University Press, 1950).
3. Robert Sampson and John Laub, *Crime in the Making: Pathways and Turning Points Through Life* (Cambridge: Harvard University Press, 1993). According to Sampson and Laub, the Gluecks' work has never been "well integrated into modern criminological theory and research" (37). One reason, they suggest, is that the Gluecks were never fully accepted in academia and were generally considered outcasts. Their outlook was interdisciplinary and was not beholden to any particular discipline. This was unfortunate, since the Gluecks collected an impressive set of data that demonstrates clearly what happens to juvenile delinquents.
4. Ibid., 136.
5. Lee N. Robins, *Deviant Children Grown Up* (Baltimore: Williams & Wilkins, 1966).
6. Ibid., 32.
7. Terrie Moffit, "Adolescence-limited and life-course-persistent antisocial behavior: a developmental taxonomy," *Psychological Review* 100 (1993): 674–701.
8. Richard L. Jenkins had a longstanding interest in the classification of delinquent behavior and strongly believed that degree of socialization was important in determining a patient's ultimate outcome. Fritz A. Henn, Rebecca Bardwell, and Jenkins reported that 58% of 62 socialized delinquents but only 37% of 19 undersocialized aggressive delinquents had no subsequent convictions. See "Juvenile delinquents revisited: adult criminal activity," *Archives of General Psychiatry* 37 (1980): 1160–1163.

9. In 1977, the Maryland legislature abolished the indeterminate sentence. The Patuxent experience is described by Bridget Dolan and Jeremy Coid in *Psychopathic and Antisocial Personality Disorder: Treatment and Research Issues* (London: Gaskell, 1993), 199–203.

10. Dr. Charles Shagass, a psychiatrist at the University of Iowa in the 1960s, thought that LSD and related drugs could facilitate insight and induce periods of remission from antisocial behavior. For information regarding his studies, see Roy Edward Wilson and Charles Shagass, "Comparison of two drugs with psychotomimetic effects (LSD and Ditran)," *Journal of Nervous and Mental Diseases* 138 (1964): 277–286; and Charles Shagass and Robert M. Bittle, "Therapeutic effects of LSD: a follow-up study," *Journal of Nervous and Mental Diseases* 144 (1967): 471–478.

11. Robins, *Deviant Children Grown Up*, 221–237.

12. See Donald W. Black, Connie H. Baumgard, and Sue E. Bell, "A 16- to 45-year follow-up of 41 males with antisocial personality disorder," *Comprehensive Psychiatry* 36 (1995): 130–140; Black, Baumgard, and Bell, "A long-term outcome of antisocial personality disorder compared with depression, schizophrenia, and surgical conditions," *Bulletin of the American Academy of Psychiatry and the Law* 23 (1995): 43–52; and Black, Baumgard, Bell, and Chi Kao, "Death rates in 71 subjects with antisocial personality disorder compared with general population mortality," *Psychosomatics* 37 (1996): 131–136.

13. Robins, *Deviant Children Grown Up*, 236.

14. Robins, "The Epidemiology of Antisocial Personality," in *Psychiatry*, Volume 3, Chapter 19, eds. Robert O. Michels and Jesse O. Cavenar (Philadelphia: J. B. Lippincott, 1987), 12. A study of elderly offenders is reported by L. J. Epstein, C. Mills, and A. Simon in "Antisocial behavior of the elderly," *Comprehensive Psychiatry* 11 (1970): 36–42.

15. See Robins, *Deviant Children Grown Up*, 229–237; and Donald W. Black, Patrick Monahan, Connie H. Baumgard, and Sue E. Bell, "Predictors of long-term outcome in 45 men with antisocial personality disorder," *Annals of Clinical Psychiatry* 9 (1997): 211–217.

16. Sampson and Laub, *Crime in the Making*, 135–138.

17. See S. Alexandra Burt, Brent Donnellan, Mikhila N. Humbad, et al., "Does marriage inhibit antisocial behavior? An examination of selection vs causation via a longitudinal twin design," *Archives of General Psychiatry* 67 (2010): 1309–1315.

18. The fact that antisocials frequently develop other psychiatric disorders is well documented. Mark Zimmerman and William Coryell assessed 26 antisocials and found that 12% had a history of mania, 35% a history of major depression, 77% a history of alcohol abuse/dependence, 54% a history of drug abuse/dependence, 27% a history of phobic disorder, and 39% a history of psychosexual dysfunction. See "DSM-III personality disorder diagnoses in a nonpatient sample," *Archives of General Psychiatry* 46 (1989): 682–689. Using ECA

study data, Jeffrey H. Boyd, Jack D. Burke, Jr., Ernest Gruenberg, et al., showed a clear relationship between ASP and major depression, alcohol abuse/dependence, obsessive-compulsive disorder (OCD), phobias, and panic disorder. See "Exclusion criteria of DSM-III: a study of co-occurrence of hierarchy-free syndromes," *Archives of General Psychiatry* 41 (1988): 983–989. More recent data come from the NESARC study, which verifies the relationship of ASP to other comorbid disorders. See William M. Compton, Kevin P. Conway, Frederick S. Stinson, et al., "Prevalence, correlates, and comorbidity of DSM-IV antisocial personality syndromes and alcohol and specific drug use disorders in the United States: results from the National Epidemiologic Survey on Alcohol and Related Conditions," *Journal of Clinical Psychiatry* 66 (2005): 677–685.

19. In the ECA study, antisocials were nearly 30 times more likely than non-antisocial individuals to have any type of substance use disorder. They were 21 times more likely to show alcohol abuse/dependence and 13 times more likely to show drug abuse/dependence. See Darrell A. Regier, Mary E. Farmer, Donald S. Rae, et al., "Comorbidity of mental disorders with alcohol and other drug abuse: results from the Epidemiologic Catchment Area study," *Journal of the American Medical Association* 264 (1990): 2511–2518. For data from the recent NESARC study, see Compton, Conway, Stinson, et al., cited above.

20. See Stephen H. Dinwiddie and Theodore Reich, "Attribution of antisocial symptoms in coexistent antisocial personality disorder and substance abuse," *Comprehensive Psychiatry* 34 (1993): 235–242.

21. The relationships among gambling, alcoholism, and ASP is described by Henry R. Lesieur, Sheila B. Blume, and Richard M. Zoppa in "Alcoholism, drug abuse and gambling," *Alcoholism: Clinical and Experimental Research* 10 (1986): 33–38. In a study of 140 drug-abusing antisocials, Risë B. Goldstein, Sally I. Powers, Jane McCusker, et al. reported that 29% were pathological gamblers. See "Lack of remorse in antisocial personality disorder among drug abusers in residential treatment," *Journal of Personality Disorders* 10 (1996): 321–334. In my own work, I have reported that 15% to 40% of pathological (compulsive) gamblers are antisocial. See Tami Argo and Donald W. Black, "The Characteristics of Pathological Gambling," in *Understanding and Treating Pathological Gambling*, eds. Jon E. Grant and Marc N. Potenza (Washington, D.C., American Psychiatric Publishing, Inc., 2004), 39–54.

22. Mark Zimmerman and William Coryell found that 15% of 26 antisocials had attempted suicide compared with 2% of people with no personality disorder, in "DSM-III personality disorder diagnoses in a non-patient sample," *Archives of General Psychiatry* 46 (1989): 682–689. Recent data from the United Kingdom yield very similar figures. Simone Ullrich and Jeremy Coid found that 18% of antisocials had attempted suicide compared with 4% of the rest of the population. See "Antisocial personality disorder: co-morbid Axis I mental disorders and health service use among a national household population," *Personality and*

Mental Health 3 (2009): 151–164. Michael J. Garvey and Frank Spoden discuss the meaning of suicide attempts among antisocials in "Suicide attempts in antisocial personality disorder," *Comprehensive Psychiatry* 21 (1980): 146–149. They found that 72% of 39 antisocials admitted to the St. Paul-Ramsey Medical Center had made a total of 63 previous suicide attempts, but only three of them required two or more days of hospitalization. They point out that antisocials tend to use nonviolent means that do not produce medically serious injuries, supporting their hypothesis that antisocials use suicide attempts to manipulate others or to act out their frustration.

23. Rachel Gittelman, Salvatore Mannuzza, Ronald Shanker, and Noreen Bonagura, "Hyperactive boys almost grown up: I. Psychiatric status," *Archives of General Psychiatry* 42 (1985): 937–947; Salvatore Mannuzza, Rachel Gittelman-Klein, Paula Horowitz-Konig, and Tina Louise Giampino, "Hyperactive boys almost grown up: IV. Criminality and its relationship to psychiatric status," *Archives of General Psychiatry* 46 (1989): 1073–1079; and Salvatore Mannuzza, Rachel G. Klein, Abrah Bessler, et al., "Adult outcome of hyperactive boys: educational achievement, occupational rank, and psychiatric status," *Archives of General Psychiatry* 50 (1993): 565–576. These papers draw on the same study and show the overlap between ADHD and ASP.

24. In *Deviant Children Grown Up*, Robins showed that antisocials were more likely than controls to report unexplained physical complaints (122). The relationship of ASP to somatization disorder is further explored in the following papers: C. Robert Cloninger and Samuel B. Guze, "Female criminals: their personal, familial, and social backgrounds," *Archives of General Psychiatry* 23 (1970): 554–558; Samuel B. Guze, Robert A. Woodruff, and Paula J. Clayton, "Hysteria and antisocial behavior: further evidence of an association," *American Journal of Psychiatry* 127 (1971): 957–960; and Scott Lilienfeld, "The association between antisocial personality disorder and somatization disorders: a review and integration of theoretical models," *Clinical Psychology Review* 12 (1992): 641–662.

25. See M. Orne, D. F. Dinges, and E. C. Orbe, "On the differential diagnosis of multiple personality in the forensic context," *International Journal of Experimental Hypnosis* 32 (1984): 118–169.

26. Marc D. Feldman, Charles V. Ford, and Toni Reinhold, *Patient or Pretender: Inside the Strange World of Factitious Disorders* (New York: John Wiley & Sons, 1993), 190.

27. The link between paraphilias and ASP is described by Gene G. Abel, Joanne L. Rouleau, and Jerry Cunningham-Rathner, "Sexually Aggressive Behavior," *Forensic Psychiatry and Psychology*, eds. J. Curran, A. Louis McGarry, and Salleem A. Shah (Philadelphia: F. A. Davis, 1986), 289–313; Linda S. Grossman and James L. Cavenaugh, "Psychopathology and denial in alleged sex offenders," *Journal of Nervous and Mental Disease* 178 (1990): 739–744; and Susan L. McElroy, Cesar A. Soutullo, Purcell Taylor, Jr., et al., "Psychiatric features of

36 men convicted of sexual offenses," *Journal of Clinical Psychiatry* 60 (1999): 441–420.

28. See Ronald Bayer, *Homosexuality and American Psychiatry: The Politics of Diagnosis* (New York: Basic Books, 1981).

29. At the federal level, the Sexual Offender (Jacob Wetterling) Act of 1994 requires persons convicted of sex crimes against children to notify local law enforcement of any change of address or employment after release from custody (prison or psychiatric facility). See also "Court Upholds Megan's Law in Split Ruling," *New York Times*, August 21, 1997.

30. "Natural Born Predators," *U.S. News and World Report*, September 19, 1994, 65–73.

31. "Sexual Predator Ruling Raises Ethical, Moral Dilemma," *Psychiatric Times*, August 1997.

6. Seeds of Despair

1. Harry Lionel Shapiro, *Migration and Environment* (New York: Oxford University Press, 1939).

2. "Eustaquio Deases Describes His Drug-driven Lifestyle," *Des Moines Register*, April 9, 1990.

3. See Samuel B. Guze, Edwin D. Wolfgram, Joe McKinney, and Dennis Cantwell, "Psychiatric illness in the relatives of convicted criminals: a study of 519 first-degree relatives," *Diseases of the Nervous System* 28 (1967): 651–659. A companion study of female criminals was reported by C. Robert Cloninger and Samuel Guze, "Psychiatric illness in the families of female criminals: a study of 280 first-degree relatives," *British Journal of Psychiatry* 122 (1973): 697–703. A more recent study with similar findings was reported by Stephen H. Dinwiddie and Theodore Reich, "Attribution of antisocial symptoms in co-existent antisocial personality disorder and substance abuse," *Comprehensive Psychiatry* 34 (1993): 235–242. Using a relatively broad definition of ASP, Dinwiddie and Reich found that 29% of 364 first-degree relatives were alcoholic, 28% suffered depression, 25% were drug dependent, 15% had ASP, and 4% had somatization disorder. In my own study, 17% of first-degree relatives had ASP and 26% were alcoholic—figures much higher than what would be expected in the general population (about 3.5% and 12%, respectively). Broken down by gender, 24% of male relatives and 12% of female relatives were antisocial.

4. Patricia A. Brennen and Sarnoff A. Mednick, "Genetic perspectives on crime," *Acta Psychiatrica Scandinavica*, supplement 370 (1993): 19–26.

5. Raymond Crowe, "An adoption study of antisocial personality," *Archives of General Psychiatry* 31 (1974): 784–791.

6. The remarkable Danish Adoption Study has helped to change the way we think of many psychiatric illnesses—especially schizophrenia—and the data for antisocial behavior show the influence of genetic transmission. The study is described in *The Transmission of Schizophrenia*, eds. Seymour S. Kety and David Rosenthal (Oxford: Pergamon Press, 1968). Data from the study also are reported by Fini Schulsinger in "Psychopathy: heredity and environment," *International Journal of Mental Health* 1 (1972): 190–206; and by Sarnoff A. Mednick, William F. Gabrielli, and Barry Hutchings, "Genetic influences in criminal convictions: evidence from an adoption cohort," *Science* 224 (1984): 891–894.

7. See Remi Cadoret, Thomas O'Gorman, Edward Troughton, and Ellen Heywood, "Alcoholism and antisocial personality: interrelationships, genetic, and environmental factors," *Archives of General Psychiatry* 42 (1985): 161–167; and Remi Cadoret, Edward Troughton, and Thomas O'Gorman, "Genetic and environmental factors in alcohol abuse and antisocial personality," *Journal of the Study of Alcoholism* 48 (1987): 1–8. Cadoret's initial work was reported in "Psychopathology in adopted away offspring of biologic parents with antisocial behavior," *Archives of General Psychiatry* 35 (1978): 167–184; and in Remi J. Cadoret, William R. Yates, Ed Troughton, et al., "Genetic-environment interaction in the genesis of aggressivity and conduct disorders," *Archives of General Psychiatry* 52 (1995): 916–924.

8. Wendy Slutske provides a comprehensive review on genetic transmission in "The genetics of antisocial behavior," *Current Psychiatry Reports* 3 (2001): 158–162.

9. Marie Åsberg, Lil Träskman, and Peter Thoren, "5-HIAA in the cerebrospinal fluid: a biochemical suicide predictor?" *Archives of General Psychiatry* 33 (1976): 1193–1197.

10. Matti Virkunen, Arto Nuutila, Frederick K. Goodwin, et al., "Cerebrospinal fluid monoamine metabolite levels in male arsonists," *Archives of General Psychiatry* 44 (1987): 241–247. See also Gerald L. Brown, Frederick K. Goodwin, James C. Ballenger, et al., "Aggression in humans: correlates with CSF monoamines," *Psychiatry Research* 1 (1979): 131–139.

11. See F. Gerald Moeller, Donald M. Dougherty, Alan C. Swann, et al., "Tryptophan depletion and aggressive responding in healthy males," *Psychopharmacology* 126 (1996): 97–103; and Victor Molina, Lucien Ciesielski, Serge Gobaille, et al., "Inhibition of mouse killing behavior by serotonin-mimetic drugs: effects of partial alterations of serotonin neurotransmission," *Pharmacology, Biochemistry, and Behavior* 27 (1987): 123–131. See also Marguerite Vergnes, Antoine Depaulis, and Annie Boehrer, "Parachlorophenylalanine-induced serotonin depletion increases offensive but not defensive aggression in male rats," *Physiology and Behavior* 36 (1986): 653–658; and Maurizio Fava, Jonathan Alpert, Andrew A. Nierenberg, et al., "Fluoxetine treatment of anger attacks: a replication study," *Annals of Clinical Psychiatry* 8 (1996): 7–10. Summaries of the serotonin-aggression connection are provided by Larry J. Siever and Kenneth L. Davis

in "A psychobiological perspective on the personality disorders," *American Journal of Psychiatry* 148 (1991): 1647–1658; and by Enrique S. Garza-Trevino in "Neurobiological factors in aggressive behavior," *Hospital and Community Psychiatry* 45 (1994): 690–699.

12. Peter D. Kramer, *Listening to Prozac* (New York: Viking Penguin, 1993), 134.

13. Avshalom Caspi, J. McClay, Terrie E. Moffitt, et al., "Role of genotype in the cycle of violence in maltreated children," *Science* 297 (2002): 851–854; see also Debra L Foley, Lindon J. Eaves, Brandon Wormley, et al., "Childhood adversity, monoamine oxidase A genotype and risk for conduct disorder," *Archives of General Psychiatry* 61 (2004): 738–744; and Robert A. Philibert, Pamela Wernett, Jeff Plume, et al., "Gene environment interaction with novel variable *Monoamine Oxidase* A transcriptional enhancer are associated with antisocial personality disorder," *Biological Psychiatry* 87 (2011): 366–371. In the paper by Foley and colleagues, children with a low-activity variant of MAOA were found to be at increased for risk of conduct disorder in the presence of abuse; the paper from Philibert and colleagues confirmed the findings of Caspi et al. in women.

14. The role of dopamine is explored by Michael J. Minzenberg and Larry J. Siever in "Neurochemistry and Pharmacology of Psychopathy and Related Disorders," in *Handbook of Psychopathy*, ed. Christopher J. Patrick (New York: Guilford, 2006), 251–277.

15. See John Archer, "Testosterone and aggression," in *The Psychobiology of Aggression*, eds. Marc Hillebrand and Nathaniel J. Pallone (New York: Haworth, 1994), 3–26; Howard G. Gottesman and Daniel S. P. Schubert, "Low-dose oral medroxyprogesterone acetate in the management of the paraphilias," *Journal of Clinical Psychiatry* 54 (1993): 182–188; and Martin P. Kafka, "Current concepts in the drug treatment of paraphilias and paraphilia-related disorders," *CNS Drugs* 3 (1995): 9–21. Anabolic steroids are widely abused by athletes, who have been reported to develop a broad range of psychiatric complications. See Harrison G. Pope and David L. Katz, "Homicide and near homicide by anabolic steroid users," *Journal of Clinical Psychiatry* 51 (1990): 28–31; Paul. J. Perry, William R. Yates, and Kent H. Anderson, "Psychiatric symptoms associated with anabolic steroids—a controlled, retrospective study," *Annals of Clinical Psychiatry* 2 (1990): 11–17; and Athanasios Maras, Manfred Laucht, Dirk Gerdes, et al., "Association of testosterone and dihydrotestosterone with externalizing behavior in adolescent boys and girls," *Psychoneuroendocrinology* 28 (2003): 932–940.

16. The relationship of diet and hypoglycemia to violent behavior is reviewed by Adrian Raine in *The Psychopathology of Crime* (New York: Academic Press, 1993), 209–211; William Davies, "Violence in Prisons," in *Developments in the Study of Criminal Behavior*, Volume 2, *Violence*, ed. Philip Feldman (London: John Wiley & Sons, 1982); and by Sara Solnick and David Hemenway in "The 'Twinkie Defense': The relationship between carbonated non-diet

soft drinks and violence perpetration among Boston high school students," *Injury Prevention*, published online October 24, 2011. DOI:10.1136/injuryprev-2011-040117.

17. Stephen J. Schoenthaler, "The effect of sugar on the treatment and control of antisocial behavior: a double-blind study of an incarcerated juvenile population," *International Journal of Biosocial Research* 3 (1982): 1–9.

18. Because EEGs were one of the few medical tests available in the 1940s and 1950s, they were commonly used in evaluating patients, including delinquent children and antisocial adults. Richard L. Jenkins, who later became head of child psychiatry at the University of Iowa, wrote about this with colleague Bernard L. Pacella in "Electroencephalographic studies of delinquent boys," *American Journal of Orthopsychiatry* 13 (1943): 107–120. John R. Knott, another faculty member at the University of Iowa, showed with colleagues Eleanor B. Platt, M. Coulson Ashby, and Jacques S. Gottlieb, that abnormal EEGs were common in "psychopathic personality" and their relatives, in "A familial evaluation of the electroencephalogram of patients with primary behavior disorder and psychopathic personality," *EEG Clinics in Neurophysiology* 5 (1953): 363–370.

19. Antonio Damasio, *Descartes' Error: Emotion, Reason, and the Human Brain* (New York: Grossett/Putnam, 1994), 3–10.

20. Hanna Damasio, Thomas Grabowski, Randall Frank, et al., "The return of Phineas Gage: clues about the brain from the skull of a famous patient," *Science* 264 (1994): 1102–1105.

21. Jordan Grafman, Karen Schwab, Deborah Warden, et al., "Frontal lobe injuries, violence, and aggression: a report of the Vietnam head injury study," *Neurology* 46 (1996): 1231–1238. See also Daniel Tranel, Antoine Bechara, and Natalie L. Denberg, "Asymmetric functional roles of right and left ventromedial prefrontal cortices in social conduct, decision-making, and emotional processing," *Cortex* 38 (2002): 589–612; and Mario F. Mendez, Andrew K. Chen, Jill S. Shapira, and Bruce L. Miller, "Acquired sociopathy and frontotemporal dementia," *Dementia and Geriatric Cognitive Disorders* 20 (2005): 99–104.

22. Terrie E. Moffitt reviews evidence supporting developmental theories of antisocial behavior in "Adolescence-limited and life-course-persistent antisocial behavior: a developmental taxonomy," *Psychological Review* 100 (1993): 674–701; and in "The neuropsychology of conduct disorder," *Development and Psychopathology* 5 (1993): 135–151.

23. Lauren S. Wakschlag, Benjamin B. Lahey, Rolf Loeber, et al. found that maternal smoking was an important risk factor for the development of conduct disorder and hypothesized that smoking reduces the oxygen supply to the developing fetal brain. The findings are reported in "Maternal smoking during pregnancy and its risk of conduct disorder in boys," *Archives of General Psychiatry* 54 (1997): 670–676.

24. See Peter Goyer, Paul Andreasen, Anita Clayton, et al., "Positron-emission tomography and personality disorder," *Neuropsychopharmacology* 10 (1994): 21–28.

25. Adrian Raine is one of the most innovative leaders in the quest to understand the neural basis of antisocial and psychopathic behavior. See Adrian Raine, Monte S. Buchsbaum, and Lori LaCasse, "Brain abnormalities in murderers indicated by positron emission tomography," *Biological Psychiatry* 42 (1997): 495–508; Adrian Raine, Todd Lencz, Susan Bihrle, et al., "Reduced prefrontal gray matter volume and reduced autonomic activity in antisocial personality disorder," *Archives of General Psychiatry* 57 (2000): 119–127; Yaling Yang, Adrian Raine, Katharine L. Narr, et al., "Localisation of prefrontal white matter in pathological liars," *British Journal of Psychiatry* 190 (2007): 174–175; and Yaling Yang, Adrian Raine, Katharine L. Narr, et al., "Localization of deformations within the amygdala of individuals with psychopathy," *Archives of General Psychiatry* 66 (2009): 986–994. For reviews of brain imaging research in antisocials, see Yaling Yang, Andrea L. Glenn, and Adrian Raine, "Brain abnormalities in antisocial individuals: implications for the law," *Behavioral Sciences and the Law* 26 (2008): 65–83; and Mairead C. Dolan, "What imaging tells us about violence in anti-social men," *Criminal Behavior and Mental Health* 20 (2010): 199–214.

26. See Kent A. Kiehl, Andra M. Smith, Robert D. Hare, et al., "Limbic abnormalities in affective processing by criminal psychopaths as revealed by functional magnetic resonance imaging," *Biological Psychiatry* 50 (2001): 677–684; and Kent A. Kiehl, A. M. Smith, A. Mendrek, et al., "Temporal lobe abnormalities in semantic processing by criminal psychopaths as revealed by functional magnetic resonance imaging," *Psychiatry Research: Neuroimaging* 130 (2004): 27–42. For an interesting profile of Kiehl's work, see Greg Miller's "Investigating the Psychopathic Mind," in *Science* 321 (2008): 1284–1286.

27. The psychophysiological theory of psychopathic behavior is discussed by Robert Hare in "Electrodermal and Cardiovascular Correlates of Psychopathy," in *Psychopathic Behavior: Approaches to Research*, eds. Robert D. Hare and Daisy Schalling (New York: John Wiley & Sons, 1978), 107–144. See also Mairead Dolan, "Psychopathy: a neurobiologic perspective," *British Journal of Psychiatry* 115 (1994): 151–159.

28. The possible significance of abnormal psychophysiologic measures is discussed by Angela Scarpa and Adrain Raine in "Psychophysiology of anger and violent behavior," *Psychiatric Clinics of North America* 20 (1997): 375–403.

29. See Hans J. Eysenck, "Is conscience a conditioned reflex?" in *Crime and Personality*, revised ed. (London: Routledge and Kegan Paul, 1977), 105–129, esp. 118–119.

30. Raine, *The Psychopathology of Crime*, 178–180.

31. See Adrian Raine, Peter H. Venables, and Mark Williams, "Relationships between central and autonomic measures of arousal at age 15 years and criminality at age 24 years," *Archives of General Psychiatry* 47 (1990): 1003–1007.

32. Lee N. Robins, *Deviant Children Grown Up* (Baltimore: Williams & Wilkins, 1966), 182–189.

33. Sheldon Glueck and Eleanor Glueck, *Unraveling Juvenile Delinquency* (Cambridge: Harvard University Press, 1950), 163.

34. John Bowlby, *Forty-Four Juvenile Thieves: Their Character and Home-life* (Baillere, England: Tindall and Cox, 1946); Michael Rutter, *Maternal Deprivation Reassessed*, 2nd ed. (Harmondsworth, England: Penguin, 1982).

35. For a discussion of the effect of divorce or separation on antisocial behavior, see Raine, *The Psychopathology of Crime*, 252–257.

36. Ibid., 259–260.

37. See Rolf Loeber, "Development and risk factors of juvenile antisocial behavior and delinquency," *Clinical Psychology Review* 10 (1990): 1–41.

38. See Lee Ellis, "The victimful-victimless crime distinction and seven universal demographic correlates of victimful crime behavior," *Personality and Individual Differences* 9 (1988): 528–548.

39. Jack Abbott, *In the Belly of the Beast* (New York: Vintage, 1981), 108.

40. Glueck and Glueck, *Unraveling Juvenile Delinquency*, 163.

41. See Kenneth A. Dodge, Joseph M. Price, Jo-Anne Bachorowski, and Joseph P. Newman "Hostile attributional biases in severely aggressive adolescents," *Journal of Abnormal Psychology* 99 (1990): 388–392.

42. Jaana Juvonen and Alice Ho, "Social motives underlying antisocial behavior across middle school grades," *Journal of Youth and Adolescence* 37 (2008): 747–756.

43. Leon Bing, *Do or Die* (New York: HarperPerennial, 1991), 12.

44. Rolf Loeber, Magda Strouthamer-Loeber, and Stephanie M. Green, "Age at onset of problem behavior in boys and later disruptive and delinquent behaviors," *Criminal Behavior and Mental Health* 1 (1991): 229–246.

45. See Barbara K. Luntz and Cathy Spatz Widom, "Antisocial personality disorder in abused and neglected children grown up," *American Journal of Psychiatry* 101 (1994): 670–674. See also V. E. Pollock, John Briere, Lon Schneider, et al., "Childhood antecedents of antisocial behavior: parental alcoholism and physical abusiveness," *American Journal of Psychiatry* 147 (1990): 1290–1293; and Jeffrey G. Johnson, Patricia Cohen, Jocelyn Brown, et al., "Childhood maltreatment increases risk of personality disorders during early childhood," *Archives of General Psychiatry* 56 (1999): 600–606.

46. Adrian Raine, Patricia Brennan, and Sarnoff A. Mednick, "Birth complications combined with early maternal rejection at age 1 year predisposes to violent crime at age 18 years," *Archives of General Psychiatry* 51 (1994): 584–988.

47. An intriguing theory of how abuse alters brain structure is considered by J. Douglas Bremner, John H. Krystal, Dennis Charney, and Steven M. Southwick in "Neural mechanisms in dissociative amnesia for childhood abuse: relevance to the current controversy surrounding 'false memory syndrome,'" *American Journal of Psychiatry* 153 (1996): 71–82; and by Dorothy Otnow Lewis in "From abuse to violence: psychological consequences of maltreatment," *Journal of the American Academy of Child and Adolescent Psychiatry* 31 (1992): 383–391.

48. See L. Rowell Huesmann, Jessica F. Moise, and Cheryl-Lynn Podolski, "The Effects of Media Violence on the Development of Antisocial Behavior," in *Handbook of Antisocial Behavior*, eds. David M. Stoff, James Breiling, and John Maser (New York: John Wiley & Sons, 1997) 181–193; and L. Rowell Huesmann and Laramie D. Taylor, "The role of media violence in violent behavior," *Annual Review of Public Health* 27 (2006): 393–415.

7. Overcoming Antisocial Personality Disorder

1. Antisocials are problem patients in hospitals, as Francis L. Carney discusses in "Inpatient Treatment Programs," in *The Psychopath: A Comprehensive Study of Antisocial Disorders and Behaviors*, ed. William H. Reid (New York: Brunner/ Mazel, 1978), 261–285. See also William H. Reid, "The antisocial personality: a review," *Hospital and Community Psychiatry* 36 (1985): 831–837.

2. William and Joan McCord, *Psychopathy and Delinquency* (New York: Grune & Stratton, 1956), 84.

3. For a discussion of countertransference, see Larry H. Strasburger, "The Treatment of Antisocial Syndromes: The Therapist's Feelings," in *Unmasking the Psychopath: Antisocial Personality and Related Syndromes*, eds. William H. Reid, Darwin Dorr John I. Walker, and Jack W. Bonner (New York: W. W. Norton, 1986), 191–207; Aaron Beck, Arthur Freeman, and Denise D. Davis, et al., "Antisocial Personality Disorder," in *Cognitive Therapy of Personality Disorders, Second Edition* (New York: Guilford Press, 2006), 162–186; and W. H. Reid, "The antisocial personality: a review," *Hospital and Community Psychiatry* 36 (1985): 831–837. A more recent discussion of the problems encountered in treating antisocials will be found in an article by Kate Davidson, Judith Halford, Lindsay Kirkwood, et al.; they describe the difficulties faced by patients and therapists in "CBT for violent men with antisocial personality disorder: reflections on the experience of carrying out therapy in MASCOT, a pilot randomized controlled trial," *Personality and Mental Health* 4 (2010): 86–95.

4. Hervey Cleckley, *The Mask of Sanity: An Attempt to Clarify Some Issues About the So-called Psychopathic Personality*, 5th ed. (St. Louis: C. V. Mosby, 1976), 476–477.

5. Beck et al., *Cognitive Therapy of Personality Disorders*, Second Edition, 168. Beck's chapter on ASP discusses the various objectives of cognitive therapy with antisocials and specific interventions. He provides case examples and typical dialogue between patient and therapist.

6. Robert D. Hare, *Without Conscience—The Disturbing World of the Psychopaths Among Us* (New York: Pocket Books, 1993), 195.

7. Preliminary evidence of the effectiveness of cognitive behavioral therapy in ASP includes a study of opiate addicts treated in a methadone maintenance program reported by George E. Woody, A. Thomas McLellan, Lester Luborsky, and Charles P. O'Brien in "Sociopathy and psychotherapy outcome," *Archives of General Psychiatry* 42 (1985): 1081–1086. The researchers noted that subjects with ASP and major depression responded well to cognitive therapy or supportive-expressive psychotherapy. Improvement included a reduction in drug use, illegal activity, and psychiatric symptoms. Kate M. Davidson and Peter Tyrer used cognitive therapy to treat ASP and reported that two of three antisocials engaged in treatment and improved in target problem areas. See "Cognitive therapy for antisocial and borderline personality disorders: single case study series," *British Journal of Clinical Psychology* 35 (1996): 413–429. Recently, Kate Davidson, Peter Tyrer, Philip Tata, et al. have further explored CBT in antisocial men, and, although the trial did not show CBT more effective than "usual care," the authors pointed out that it wasn't a fair test of CBT because of the small sample size and low statistical power. See "CBT for violent men with antisocial personality disorder in the community: an exploratory randomized controlled trial," *Psychological Medicine* 39 (2009): 569–577. The National Institute for Health and Clinical Excellence (NICE) in the United Kingdom concludes that evidence supporting psychotherapy for ASP is limited, but that evidence supports group-based cognitive behavioral therapy for reducing reoffending behavior in antisocials with coexisting substance abuse, and for reducing reoffending behavior in adults and adolescents in criminal justice settings. NICE recommends treatment of coexisting substance misuse, depression, and anxiety. For the full report, see NICE (2009), "Antisocial personality disorder: treatment, management and prevention," in *Clinical Guideline* 77. London: NICE. Retrieved March 20, 2012, from http://www.nice.org.uk/guidance/CG77.

8. Gabbard lectured at the 2003 American Psychiatric Association Institute on Psychiatric Services, held in Boston, Massachusetts. See Mark Moran, "Antisocial personality disorder: when is it treatable?," *Psychiatric News*, January 2, 2004.

9. The lack of research makes it difficult to make medication recommendations. I and others have had to extrapolate from the literature on the treatment of aggressive or disruptive behaviors in other patient groups, such as kids with conduct disorder, brain injured or dementia patients, psychotic patients, or

those with borderline personality disorder. In a telling review, performed for the authoritative Cochrane Collaborative, Najat Khalifa, Connor Duggan, Jutta Stoffers, et al. conclude the following: "The body of evidence ... is insufficient to allow any conclusion to be drawn about the use of pharmacologic interventions in the treatment of antisocial personality disorder." See "Pharmacologic interventions for antisocial personality disorder," *Cochrane Database of Systematic Reviews* 8 (2010): DOI: 10:1002/14651858CD007667.pub2. In the NICE review, cited above, it was concluded that data was insufficient to recommend the routine use of medication for ASP, and that medication for coexisting disorders should follow relevant clinical guidelines for the condition in question.

10. The use of lithium to reduce aggression in prisoners is well documented. See Michael H. Sheard, "Effect of lithium in human aggression," *Nature* 230 (1971): 113–114. Twelve young men with impulsive and aggressive behaviors improved with lithium. Sheard and colleagues James L. Marini, Carolyn I. Bridges, and Ernest Wagner then carried out a double-blind study reported in "The effect of lithium on impulsive aggressive behavior in man," *American Journal of Psychiatry* 133 (1976): 1409–1413. All 80 subjects had been convicted of aggressive crimes, including murder, rape, and manslaughter. Those who received lithium experienced a significant drop in the number of serious infractions while in prison (e.g., threatening behavior, actual assaults) compared with those who received a placebo. In "Lithium in hospitalized aggressive children with conduct disorder: a double-blind and placebo-controlled trial," *Journal of the American Academy of Child and Adolescent Psychiatry* 34 (1995): 445–453, Magda Campbell and colleagues reported that lithium demonstrated an "antiaggression specificity" and was superior to placebo. The presence of hyperactivity contributed to a favorable response. See Ernest S. Barrett, Thomas A. Kent, Stephen G. Bryant, and Alan R. Felthaus, "A controlled trial of phenytoin in impulsive aggression," *Journal of Clinical Psychopharmacology* 11 (1991): 388–389; and E. S. Barrett, Matthew S. Stanford, A. R. Felthaus, and T. A. Kent, "The effects of phenytoin on impulsive and premeditated aggression: a controlled study," *Journal of Clinical Psychopharmacology* 17 (1997): 341–349. In the latter report, inmates were randomly given low doses of phenytoin or a placebo for six weeks, then given the other agent for another six weeks. Phenytoin reduced both the frequency and the intensity of impulsive aggressive acts. The drug did not reduce premeditated aggression.

11. Many reports document the effect of medication in calming aggressive behavior, and the following articles are representative. The anticonvulsant carbamazepine has been used with some success. See Jeffrey Mattes, Joanne Rosenberg, and Daniel Mays, "Carbamazepine versus propranolol in patients with uncontrolled rage outbursts: a random assignment study," *Psychopharmacology Bulletin* 20 (1984): 98–100; and Daniel Luchins, "Carbamazepine in psychiatric patients," *Psychopharmacology Bulletin* 20 (1984): 569–571. Sodium valproate also has

been beneficial in some aggressive patients. See James A. Wilcox, "Divalproex sodium in the treatment of aggressive behavior," *Annals of Clinical Psychiatry* 6 (1994): 17–20; and James A. Wilcox, "Divalproex sodium as a treatment for borderline personality disorder," *Annals of Clinical Psychiatry* 7 (1995): 33–37. See also Karin Tritt, Cerstine Nickel, Claas Lahmann, et al., "Lamotrigine treatment of aggression in female borderline patients: a randomized, double-blind, placebo-controlled study," *Journal of Psychopharmacology* 19 (2005): 287–291. For propranolol treatment, see Robert M. Greendike, Donald R. Kanter, Daniel B. Schuster, et al., "Propranolol treatment of assaultive patients with organic brain disease," *Journal of Nervous and Mental Disease* 174 (1986): 290–294; and Samuel Kuperman and Mark A. Stewart, "Use of propranolol to decrease aggressive outbursts in younger patients," *Psychosomatics* 28 (1987): 315–320. The antidepressant trazodone has been reported to reduce aggressive behavior. See Dale M. Simpson and Dodi Foster, "Improvement in organically-disturbed behavior with trazodone treatment," *Journal of Clinical Psychiatry* 47 (1986): 191–193; and Carlos A. Tejera and Stephen M. Saravay, "Treatment of organic personality syndrome with low dose trazodone," *Journal of Clinical Psychiatry* 56 (1995): 374–375. Buspirone has produced benefits in a few patients. See Aaron M. Levine, "Buspirone and agitation in head injury," *Brain Injury* 2 (1988): 165–167; and John Ratey, Robert Sovner, Allan Parks, and Kristin Rogentine, "Buspirone treatment of aggression and anxiety in mentally retarded patients: a multiple-baseline, placebo lead-in study," *Journal of Clinical Psychiatry* 52 (1991): 159–162.

12. Although primarily used to treat schizophrenia and other psychotic disorders, antipsychotic drugs may deter aggression. In a study of children with conduct disorders, Magda Campbell and colleagues reported that both haloperidol and lithium carbonate were superior to placebo in decreasing behavioral symptoms in 61 hospitalized children aged 5–13. See "Behavioral efficacy of haloperidol and lithium carbonate," *Archives of General Psychiatry* 41 (1984): 650–656. More recently, the antipsychotic risperidone has been studied in children; it reduces acting-out behaviors and increases prosocial behaviors. See Robert L. Findling, Michael G. Aman, Marielle Eerdekens, et al., "Long-term, open-label study of risperidone in children with severe disruptive behaviors and below average IQ," *American Journal of Psychiatry* 161 (2004): 677–684; and Magali Reyes, Jan Buitelaar, Paz Toren, et al., "A randomized, double-blind, placebo-controlled study of risperidone maintenance treatment in children and adolescents with disruptive behavior disorders," *American Journal of Psychiatry* 163 (2006): 402–410. Other reports on the benefits of antipsychotics come from literature on brain-damaged individuals, patients with dementia, or people with borderline personality disorder. See Henry Brodaty, David Ames, John Snowdon, et al., "A randomized placebo-controlled trial of risperidone for the treatment of aggression, agitation, and psychosis of dementia," *Journal of Clinical Psychiatry* 64

(2003): 134–143; and Menahem I. Krakowski, Pal Szobor, and Karen A. Nolan, "Atypical antipsychotics, neurocognitive deficits, and aggression in schizophrenic patients," *Journal of Clinical Psychopharmacology* 28 (2008): 485–493.

13. Patients with borderline personality disorder which, like ASP, is characterized by impulsivity, act out more frequently when given alprazolam, a benzodiazepine tranquilizer. See Rex W. Cowdry and David Gardner, "Pharmacotherapy of borderline personality disorder," *Archives of General Psychiatry* 45 (1988): 111–119.

14. Severe personality disorders reduce the effectiveness of treatment for most mental disorders, although no one knows why. See Donald Black, Sue Bell, James Hulbert, and Amelia Nasrallah, "The importance of Axis II in patients with major depression: a controlled study," *Journal of Affective Disorders* 14 (1988): 115–122. James H. Reich and Allen I. Green reviewed the subject in "Effect of personality disorders on outcome of treatment," *Journal of Nervous and Mental Disease* 179 (1991): 74–82. Major depression, panic disorder, and obsessive-compulsive disorder all show a poorer treatment response when the patient has a concurrent personality disorder.

15. The use of SSRIs in treating anger is reported in three studies. Robert N. Rubey, Michael R. Johnson, Naresh Emmanuel, and R. Bruce Lydiard reported that 9 of 11 persons treated with fluoxetine (Prozac) reported fewer anger attacks. See "Fluoxetine in the treatment of anger: an open clinical trial," *Journal of Clinical Psychiatry* 57 (1996): 398–401. Maurizio Fava, Jonathan Alpert, Andrew A. Nierenberg, et al. treated 64 depressed patients who reported anger attacks. Following treatment with fluoxetine (Prozac), the attacks disappeared in two-thirds of subjects. See "Fluoxetine treatment of anger attacks: a replication study," *Annals of Clinical Psychiatry* 8 (1996): 7–10. In an unrelated report, sertraline (Zoloft) was used to treat aggression and self-injurious behavior in nine mentally retarded adults, five of whom were also autistic. Eight of the nine were rated as improved. See Jessica A. Hellings, Lee Ann Kelley, William F. Gabrielli, et al., "Sertraline response in adults with mental retardation and autistic disorder," *Journal of Clinical Psychiatry* 57 (1996): 333–336.

16. Medroxyprogesterone has been used in people whose deviant sexual behavior is uncontrolled. See Howard G. Gottesman and Daniel S. P. Schubert, "Low-dose oral medroxyprogesterone acetate in the management of the paraphilias," *Journal of Clinical Psychiatry* 54 (1993): 182–188; and Fred S. Berlin and Carl Meinecke, "Treatment of sex offenders with antiandrogenic medication: conceptualization, review of treatment modalities, and preliminary findings," *American Journal of Psychiatry* 138 (1981): 601–607. The latter article also mentions the use of surgical castration, an option generally considered unacceptable in the United States.

17. Antisocial personality disorder adversely affects the treatment of alcohol and drug abuse, as shown in a small study by David B. Mather, "The role of antisocial

personality and alcohol rehabilitation treatment effectiveness," *Military Medicine* 152 (1987): 516–518. George A. Woody, A. Thomas McLellan, Lester Luborsky, and Charles P. O'Brien evaluated the treatment outcome in opiate addicts and determined that ASP alone was a negative predictor of the outcome of psychotherapy. See "Sociopathy and psychotherapy outcome," *Archives of General Psychiatry* 42 (1985): 1081–1086. The benefits of alcohol and drug treatment services for antisocials are reported by John S. Cacciola, Arthur I. Alterman, Megan J. Rutherford, and Edward Snider in "Treatment response of antisocial substance abusers," *Journal of Nervous and Mental Diseases* 183 (1996): 166–171; and by A. I. Alterman, M. J. Rutherford, J. S. Cacciola, et al. in "Response to methadone maintenance and counseling in antisocial patients with and without major depression," *Journal of Nervous and Mental Diseases* 184 (1996): 695–702. Their research shows—first in a group of alcohol- and cocaine-abusing persons, then in a group of opiate abusers—that treatment of substance abuse in antisocials is accompanied by a reduction in antisocial symptoms.

18. Incarceration is discussed by Peter Suedfeld and P. Bruce Landon in "Approaches to Treatment," in *Psychopathic Behavior: Approaches to Research*, eds. Robert D. Hare and Daisy Schalling (New York: John Wiley & Sons, 1978), 347–376. They observe that, although antisocial convicts tend to lead riots, traffic in drugs, spread the convict code, generally violate regulations, and spend much time in solitary confinement, prisons are successful at keeping the antisocial isolated from the community, "maintaining the safety of the latter at the expense of the freedom of the former" (359).

19. Alfred Blumstein and Jacqueline Cohen, "Characterizing criminal careers," *Science* 237 (1985): 985–991.

20. "Young Toughs Talk Peace," *Psychiatric News*, November 18, 1994. For a study of a similar project, see David C. Grossman, Holly J. Neckerman, Thomas D. Koepsell, et al., "Effectiveness of a violence prevention curriculum among children in elementary school: a randomized controlled trial," *Journal of the American Medical Association* 277 (1997): 1605–1611.

21. The Cambridge-Somerville Experiment is described by William McCord and Joan McCord, with Irving Kenneth Zola, in *Origins of Crime: A New Evaluation of the Cambridge-Somerville Youth Study* (New York: Columbia University Press, 1959).

22. Mark W. Lipsey, "The effect of treatment on juvenile delinquents: results from a meta-analysis," presented at a meeting sponsored by the National Institute of Mental Health for potential applicants for Research to Prevent Youth Violence, October 31–November 3, 1992, Bethesda, Maryland.

23. Don C. Gibbons describes the failed "scared straight" experiment in *Delinquent Behavior*, 3rd ed. (Englewood Cliffs, N.J.: Prentice Hall, 1981), 333–334.

24. See Waln K. Brown, Timothy P. Miller, and Richard L. Jenkins, "The favorable effect of juvenile court adjudication in delinquent youth on the first contact with the juvenile justice system," *Juvenile and Family Court Journal* 38 (1987): 21–26;

and "The fallacy of radical non-intervention," *Annals of Clinical Psychiatry* 1 (1989): 55–57.

8. Power and Pretense

1. Adam Nagourney and Abby Goodnough, "F.B.I. Manhunt for Mob Legend Ends After Tip on Companion," *New York Times*, June 24, 2011.
2. Leo Tolstoy, *Anna Karenina* (New York: W. W. Norton, 1970).
3. Alex Kelly's fugitive life is discussed by Jennet Conant, "The Fugitive Son," *Vanity Fair*, February 1996; and in "Man Who Fled to Europe Convicted in Rape Case," *Des Moines Register*, June 12, 1997.
4. "Alex Kelly: Fugitive Son on Trial," *Turning Point*, ABC network, December 5, 1996.
5. "Teenager Convicted of Murdering Parents," Associated Press, May 28, 1997.
6. The story of the Menendez brothers and their crimes is reported by Dominick Dunne in "Courtroom notebook—The Menendez murder trial," *Vanity Fair*, October 1993, 252–257, 312–317; "Menendez justice," *Vanity Fair*, March 1994; and "Three faces of evil," *Vanity Fair*, June 1996.
7. Colin Moynihan, "Italian Businessman Who Claimed Vatican Ties Is Sentenced to 54 Months in Prison," *New York Times*, October 24, 2008; see also Michael Shnayerson, "The Follieri charade," *Vanity Fair*, October 2008; and "Case File: Raffaello Follieri," episode 27, *American Greed*, CNBC network, November 20, 2011.
8. Bailey's history is reported by Patrick J. Kiger in "The horse lady vanishes," *Gentlemen's Quarterly*, May 1995; and by Howard Blum in "The horse murders," *Vanity Fair*, January 1995.
9. "NBA Suspends Sprewell for One Year," *Washington Post*, December 4, 1997; "Tyson Repents, Begs for Forgiveness," *Des Moines Register*, July 1, 1997.
10. See "Double trouble for 2pac," *Newsweek*, December 12, 1994; Robert Sam Anson, "To die like a gangsta," *Vanity Fair*, March 1997; and Ivan Solotaroff, "Gangsta life, gangsta death," *Esquire*, December 1996.
11. In *DSM-IV-TR*, adult antisocial behavior is categorized as a "V-code," which means that the condition is not attributable to a mental illness. Other V-code conditions include malingering and marital discord ("partner-relational problem" in *DSM* language).
12. Mark Seal, "Madoff's world," *Vanity Fair*, April 2009; Mark Seal, "Ruth's world," *Vanity Fair*, September 2009; and Marie Brenner, "Madoff in Manhattan," *Vanity Fair*, January 2009.
13. See Risë B. Goldstein, Deborah A. Dawson, Tulshi D. Saha, et al., "Antisocial behavioral syndromes and DSM-IV alcohol use disorders: results from the National Epidemiologic Survey on Alcohol and Related Conditions," *Alcoholism: Clinical and Experimental Research* 31 (2007): 814–828. I have

also written on this topic and reached similar conclusions. See Donald W. Black and David Braun, "Antisocial patients: a comparison of those with and without childhood conduct disorder," *Annals of Clinical Psychiatry* 10 (1998): 53–57.

9. The Antisocial Murderer

1. There are several books about Gacy, and one of the best is *Killer Clown: The John Wayne Gacy Murders* by Terry Sullivan and Peter T. Maiken (New York: Pinnacle Books, 1983). The book reviews Gacy's past, his murders, and his trial. Because his psychiatric charts were introduced in court documents, they are cited extensively and include several quotations used in this chapter. Other books are *The Man Who Killed Boys* by Clifford Linedecker (New York: St. Martin's Press, 1980) and *Buried Dreams: Inside the Mind of a Serial Killer* by Tim Cahill and Russ Ewing (New York: Bantam Books, 1986).

2. Sullivan and Maiken, *Killer Clown*, 175 and 208.

3. "John Gacy's Love Letters," *Chicago Sun Times*, February 28, 1988.

4. "Years on Death Row Almost Over for Gacy," *Des Moines Register*, May 8, 1994.

5. Sullivan and Maiken, *Killer Clown*, 271.

6. Cahill and Ewing, *Buried Dreams*, 85.

7. The most likely explanation for Gacy's spells is that they resulted from hyperventilation rather than an underlying heart condition. During an 1969 outpatient evaluation at the University of Iowa Hospital—Gacy was imprisoned at the Men's Reformatory in Anamosa, Iowa, at the time—he reported a history of fainting spells from age 15 on. Staff physician Elmer DeGowin and resident physician Howard Gross noted that the spells were relieved by breathing into a paper bag, as is typical in hyperventilation. Today, Gacy's spells would probably be diagnosed as panic attacks.

8. Cahill and Ewing, *Buried Dreams*, 365–366.

9. Gacy's early dating and sexual experiences are described in Sullivan and Maiken, *Killer Clown*, 257, and in Cahill and Ewing, *Buried Dreams*, 38–43.

10. Gacy's psychiatric evaluation at the University of Iowa is reported in detail by Sullivan and Maiken, *Killer Clown*, 270–272, and by Cahill and Ewing, *Buried Dreams*, 84–89.

11. Robert D. Hare, *Without Conscience—The Disturbing World of the Psychopaths Among Us* (New York: Pocket Books, 1993) 5.

12. See Risë B. Goldstein, Bridget F. Grant, June Ruan, et al., "Antisocial personality disorder with childhood- vs adolescence-onset conduct disorder: results from the National Epidemiologic Survey on Alcohol and Related Conditions," *Journal of Nervous and Mental Disease* 194 (2006): 667–675. Persons with childhood-onset ASP are compared with adolescent-onset cases and are found to be much more likely to bully and threaten others, use weapons, display cruelty to animals and people, and have more "violent symptoms at any age."

13. Serial killing includes three elements: the number of victims must exceed three, the killings occur at different times and places, and the motivation is either sexual or for internal psychological gratification. Nearly all serial killers are men. For more information about serial killers, see Gretchen W. Kramer, Wayne D. Lord, and Kirk Heilbrun, "Comparing single and serial homicidal offences," *Behavioral Science and the Law* 22 (2004): 325–343.

14. Michael H. Stone, *The Anatomy of Evil* (New York: Prometheus Books, 2009).

15. Panzram is profiled by Colin Wilson and Damon Wilson in *The Killers Among Us: Sex, Madness, and Mass Murder* (New York: Warner Books, 1995), 186–206.

16. James Alan Fox and Jack Levin, *Overkill: Mass Murder and Serial Killing Exposed* (New York: Plenum Press, 1994), 18.

17. Bundy's life is chronicled by Ann Rule, *The Stranger Beside Me, Newly Updated* (New York: Penguin Books, 1989); and by Stephen G. Michaud and Hugh Aynesworth, *The Only Living Witness* (New York: Linden Press, 1983).

18. Fox and Levin, *Overkill*, 42.

19. John Douglas and Mark Olshaker, *Mindhunter: Inside the FBI's Elite Serial Crime Unit* (New York: Scribner, 1995), 239–249.

20. Fox and Levin, *Overkill*, 43. See also Joel Norris, *Serial Killers* (New York: Anchor Books, 1989), 109–127.

21. See Brian Masters, "Dahmer's Inferno," *Vanity Fair*, November 1991; and Lionel Dahmer, *A Father's Story* (New York: William Morrow, 1994).

22. Fox and Levin, *Overkill*, 50.

23. See Robert H. Gollmar, *Ed Gein* (New York: Pinnacle Books, 1981).

24. Why serial killers are mostly male has puzzled criminologists for decades. The topic is taken up by Feggy Ostrosky-Solis, Alicia Velez-Garcia, Daniel Santana-Vargas, et al. in "Case report: a middle-aged female serial killer," *Journal of Forensic Science* 53 (2008): 1223–1230.

25. Aileen Wuernos' life of crime is reviewed in the following books: Michael Reynolds, *Dead Ends: The Pursuit, Conviction and Execution of Female Serial Killer Aileen Wuernos: The Damsel of Death* (New York: St. Martin's, 2003); and Sue Russell, *Lethal Intent: The Shocking True Story of One of America's Most Notorious Female Serial Killers* (New York: Pinnacle, 2002). Her last words were reported by John Zarrella, "Wuernos' Last Words: I'll Be Back," *CNN Network*, October 15, 2002.

26. Cahill and Ewing, *Buried Dreams*, 153.

27. "Years on Death Row Almost Over for Gacy," *Des Moines Register*, May 8, 1994.

28. Gacy's trial is chronicled by Sullivan and Maiken, *Killer Clown*, 285–375.

29. The expert psychiatric testimony is reviewed by Sullivan and Maiken, *Killer Clown*, 329–356; Heston's quotation appears on 344.

30. Associated Press, "Sheriff: DNA Identifies John Wayne Gacy Victim," November 30, 2011.

31. Douglas and Olshaker, *Mindhunter*, 344.

32. For more information about personality disorders and the insanity defense, see Landy F. Sparr, "Personality disorders and criminal law: an international

perspective," *Journal of the American Academy of Psychiatry and the Law* 37 (2009): 168–181; and Ralph Slovenko, "Commentary: personality disorders and criminal law," *Journal of the American Academy of Psychiatry and the Law* 37 (2009): 182–185.

10. Antisocial Personality Disorder and Families

1. Hervey Cleckley, *The Mask of Sanity: An Attempt to Clarify Some Issues About the So-called Psychopathic Personality*, 5th ed. (St. Louis: C. V. Mosby, 1976), 479.
2. Such a program is described in the following article: John Carpi, "Parent Training May Help Conduct Disorder," *Clinical Psychiatry News*, July 1996. Family therapy is further described by G. Pirooz Sholevar in "Family therapy for conduct disorders," *Child and Adolescent Psychiatric Clinics of North America* 10 (2001): 501–517.
3. Yuriko Egami, Daniel E. Ford, Shelly Greenfield, and Rosa M. Crum, "Psychiatric profile and sociodemographic characteristics of adults who report physically abusing or neglecting children," *American Journal of Psychiatry* 153 (1996): 921–928; Kristie K. Danielson, Terrie E. Moffitt, Avshalom Caspi, and Phil A. Silva, "Comorbidity between abuse of an adult and DSM-III-R mental disorders: evidence from an epidemiologic study," *American Journal of Psychiatry* 155 (1998): 131–133.
4. Mikal Gilmore, *Shot in the Heart* (New York: Doubleday, 1994), 242.
5. "Gun Seizures to Apply in Spouse Abuse Cases," *Des Moines Register*, August 28, 1994.
6. Donald G. Dutton with Susan K. Golant, *The Batterer: A Psychological Profile* (New York: Basic Books, 1995).

Epilogue

1. Lee N. Robins. "Sturdy predictors of adult antisocial behavior," *Psychological Medicine* 8 (1978): 621.
2. See Hervey Cleckley, *The Mask of Sanity: An Attempt to Clarify Some Issues About the So-called Psychopathic Personality*, 5th ed. (St. Louis: C. V. Mosby, 1976), 479.

RECOMMENDED READINGS

Many of the books and scientific papers cited throughout this book are written for an academic audience rather than for the general public. The following list presents a starting point for the reader interested in antisocial personality disorder (ASP): a mix of memoirs, journalism, and scholarly books listed alphabetically by title.

The Anatomy of Evil, Michal H. Stone (New York: Prometheus Books, 2009). Stone, one of the nation's foremost experts on personality disorders, has written a chilling (and absorbing) book on the nature of violent crime, and he describes a hierarchy of evil behavior.

Bad Men Do What Good Men Dream, Robert I. Simon (Washington, D.C.: American Psychiatric Press, 1996). Simon, a forensic psychiatrist, describes the dark side of human behavior by profiling many types of evildoers, from rapists to serial killers. Many, of course, are antisocial.

The Batterer: A Psychological Profile, Donald G. Dutton with Susan K. Golant (New York: Basic Books, 1995). The authors paint a grim picture of men who batter women. Although not all are antisocial, the insights drawn from these cases and the practical suggestions for dealing with batterers are helpful.

Before It's Too Late: Why Some Kids Get Into Trouble—And What Parents Can Do About It, Stanton E. Samenow (New York: Times Book, 1998). A psychologist and expert on criminal behavior, Samenow offers a highly useful guide to intervening with misbehaving children.

Cognitive Therapy of Personality Disorders, Second Edition, Aaron T. Beck, Arthur Freeman, and Denise D. Davis (New York: Guilford Press, 2006). Written by top experts in cognitive behavioral therapy, this revised book presents a description of the various personality disorders and treatments based on Beck's treatment model. The chapter on ASP is particularly useful.

Crime in the Making: Pathways and Turning Points Through Life, Robert J. Sampson and John H. Laub (Cambridge: Harvard University Press, 1993). This book describes results from a reanalysis of the follow-up data collected by Sheldon and Eleanor Glueck in Boston in the 1940s and 1950s. The data are still relevant for today's antisocial, and the book is well worth reading, although it is geared more toward the scientist than the lay person.

The Criminal Personality, Volume I: A Profile for Change, Samuel Yochelson and Stanton E. Samenow (New York: Jason Aronson, 1976). Written for professionals, this book details the history of the ASP diagnosis and describes the criminal's life and way of thinking. In *Volume II: The Change Process* (Northville, N.J.: Jason Aronson, 1977), the authors describe their institution-based group treatment of criminals, which follows a cognitive model.

Deviant Children Grown Up, Lee N. Robins (Baltimore: Williams & Wilkins, 1966. Reprinted in 1974 by Robert E. Krieger Publishing Company, Huntington, N.Y.). This book describes Robins' remarkable 30-year follow-up study of child guidance clinic patients. Based on this work, Robins essentially defined ASP as we now know it. This book is a must for anyone truly interested in ASP.

Do or Die, Leon Bing (New York: HarperCollins, 1991). Bing, a journalist, explores the lives of rival Los Angeles street gang members. She presents a horrifying look at their attitudes and behaviors through the eyes of members of two notorious gangs—the Crips and the Bloods.

The Handbook of Psychopathy, edited by Christopher J. Patrick (New York: Guilford, 2006). This dense book is filled with information about both ASP, psychopathy, and their overlap, but will not be easily understood by lay readers because of its academic bent. The writing style of its contributors is uneven, but the lineup of experts is impressive.

Inside the Criminal Mind, Stanton E. Samenow (New York: Times Books, 1984). This fascinating book attempts to explore the criminal mind, based on Samenow's considerable experience with criminals at St. Elizabeth's Hospital in Washington, D.C. Much of his work was presented earlier in *The Criminal Personality, Volumes I and II*, co-authored with Samuel Yochelson.

In the Belly of the Beast, Jack Henry Abbott (New York: Random House, 1981). Written by a convict, this series of essays explores prison life in no-holds-barred fashion. The way Abbott conducts his life and the thinking behind his actions reveal his antisocial personality. Abbot gives the criminal justice system the greatest share of blame for his failures but never explains why he was jailed in the first place.

The Jack Roller: A Delinquent Boy's Own Story, Clifford Shaw (Chicago: University of Chicago Press, 1930). This book—a minor classic in the sociology literature—describes "Stanley," a jack roller, that is, a robber of drunk or sleeping men, in 1920s Chicago. Stanley was reinterviewed decades later, an account that appears in the book *The Jack Roller at 70*, by the Jack Roller and Jon Snodgrass (Lexington, Mass.: Lexington Books, 1982). The follow-up is probably more interesting, as it shows the subject's continual life of misbehavior. Shaw later edited *Brothers in Crime* (Chicago: University of Chicago Press, 1938), describing the five Martin boys and their progression from juvenile delinquents to full-fledged criminals. The three books are out of print but will be found in many libraries.

The Mask of Sanity: An Attempt to Clarify Some Issues About the So-Called Psychopathic Personality, 5th ed., Hervey Cleckley (St. Louis: C. V. Mosby, 1976). This classic text is now out of print but should be available in libraries. It remains readable and interesting, but the prose and situations are dated. Cleckley presents case vignettes of typical "psychopaths" and dispels the notion that the condition only affects people in the lower social classes. Cleckley's text is still considered required reading for most psychiatrists-in-training.

The Psychopathology of Crime: Criminal Behavior as a Clinical Disorder, Adrian Raine (New York: Academic Press, 1993). This authoritative volume describes the evidence both for and against biological and environmental explanations for crime— not for ASP per se. The book is packed with information, and it is must reading for those seeking a scholarly approach to understanding antisocial behavior.

Shot in the Heart, Mikal Gilmore (New York: Doubleday, 1994). This book describes, in heart-wrenching detail, life in a home filled with antisocials. Gilmore's father was undoubtedly antisocial, as was his brother Gary, an infamous murderer executed in Utah in 1977. His mother and two other brothers also were troubled. Gilmore, a gifted writer, traces his family history in this compelling book.

Snakes in Suits—When Psychopaths Go to Work, Paul Babiak and Robert D. Hare (New York: HarperBusiness, 2007). In this disturbing book, psychologists Babiak and Hare explore psychopaths who sometimes inhabit the corporate world, the so-called "white collar" criminal. Skilled at manipulation, they can inflict considerable damage. The authors discuss ways to identify these individuals and deal with them.

Without Conscience—The Disturbing World of the Psychopaths Among Us, Robert D. Hare (New York: Pocket Books, 1993). This readable book presents interesting vignettes from Hare's own experience and the media to illustrate various types of antisocial behavior. His main focus is *psychopathy*, the extreme end of the antisocial spectrum. Hare, developer of a scale used to diagnose psychopathy, believes ASP is overly focused on criminal behavior and ignores important psychological traits.

INDEX

Note: Page numbers followed by n refer to notes.